Facial Resurfacing

EDITED BY

David J. Goldberg, MD, JD

Sanctuary Medical Aesthetic Center, Boca Raton, FL; Skin Laser & Surgery Specialists of
New York and New Jersey and Mount Sinai School of Medicine, New York, NY, USA

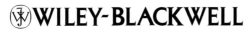

WILEY-BLACKWELL

A John Wiley & Sons, Ltd., Publication

This edition first published 2010
© 2010 Blackwell Publishing Ltd

Blackwell Publishing was acquired by John Wiley & Sons in February 2007. Blackwell's publishing program has been merged with Wiley's global Scientific, Technical and Medical business to form Wiley-Blackwell.

Registered office: John Wiley & Sons Ltd, The Atrium, Southern Gate, Chichester, West Sussex, PO19 8SQ, UK

Editorial offices: 9600 Garsington Road, Oxford, OX4 2DQ, UK
                     111 River Street, Hoboken, NJ 07030-5774, USA
                     The Atrium, Southern Gate, Chichester, West Sussex, PO19 8SQ, UK

For details of our global editorial offices, for customer services and for information about how to apply for permission to reuse the copyright material in this book please see our website at www.wiley.com/wiley-blackwell

ISBN: 978-1-4051-9080-0

A catalogue record for this book is available from the British Library.

Set in 9.5/13pt Meridien by Graphicraft Limited, Hong Kong
Printed in Singapore

1   2010

Contents

List of Contributors

Alexander L. Berlin MD
Edward E. Rotan, Jr., MD, PA, Arlington, TX, USA; Division of Dermatology, New Jersey Medical School, Newark, NJ, USA

David Beynet MD
Division of Dermatology, David Geffen School of Medicine, University of California at Los Angeles, Department of Dermatology, West Los Angeles Veteran's Administration, CA, USA

Zoe Diana Draelos MD
Consulting Professor, Department of Dermatology, Duke University School of Medicine, Durham, North Carolina, USA

Jacob Dudelzak MD
Skin Laser and Surgery Specialists of New York & New Jersey, New York, NY, USA

Timothy Corcoran Flynn MD
Cary Skin Center, Cary, NC, USA; Department of Dermatology, University of North Carolina at Chapel Hill, NC, USA

Michael H. Gold MD
Gold Skin Care Center, Tennessee Clinical Research Center, Nashville, Tennessee Clinical Assistant Professor, Vanderbilt University School of Medicine, Department of Dermatology, Vanderbilt University School of Medicine, School of Nursing, Nashville, Tennessee Visiting Professor of Dermatology, *Huashan Hospital, Fudan University*, Shanghai, China, *Number One Hospital, China Medical University*, Shenyang, China

David J. Goldberg MD, JD
Skin Laser and Surgery Specialists of New York & New Jersey, New York, NY, USA; Mount Sinai School of Medicine, New York, NY, USA; Sanctuary Medical Aesthetic Center, Boca Raton, FL, USA

Derek H. Jones MD
Division of Dermatology, David Geffen School of Medicine, University of California at Los Angeles, CA, USA

Gary D. Monheit MD
Total Skin & Beauty Dermatology Center, Birmingham, AL, USA; University of Alabama at Birmingham, Birmingham, AL, USA

Joshua A. Tournas MD
Department of Dermatology, University of California at Irvine, CA, USA

Christopher B. Zachary MBBS, FRCP
Department of Dermatology, University of California at Irvine, CA, USA

Preface

Twenty years ago facial resurfacing was accomplished with a combination of standard dermabrasion and a variety of chemical peels. With the advent of laser resurfacing, standard microdermabrasion is rarely used any more. Chemical peels, however, have not only withstood the test of time, but have become even more popular than ever. What has become clear, though, is that today's cosmetic physician ideally uses a wide variety of methods to resurface and rejuvenate the skin without surgery.

Today, facial resurfacing can lead to an exceptional cosmetic result. However, the happy patient often requires some combination of chemical peels, non-ablative laser resurfacing, fractional ablative resurfacing, non-surgical skin tightening, photodynamic therapy, dermal fillers and botulinum toxins, and cosmeceuticals. This book – with each of its seven chapters dealing with one of the aforementioned topics – ties together the complete approach to cosmetic facial resurfacing.

David J. Goldberg
New York

CHAPTER 1

Peels

Gary D. Monheit
University of Alabama at Birmingham, AL, USA

Key points
- Chemical peels remain one of the most popular and least expensive cosmetic procedures
- Peels are most easily divided by depth of penetration into superficial, medium, and deep
- The depth of peels can be generally correlated to the depth of a similar laser treatment
- Medium-depth chemical peels are the most popular physician-use peels

---

Introduction

Aging of the skin is the combined result of both intrinsic factors and extrinsic (external) influences from the environment. Intrinsic aging is the role played by genetics in relation to chronologic age. The intrinsic processes include alteration of skeletal mass and proportion, atrophy and redistribution of subcutaneous fat, increased laxity of underlying fascia and musculature, and skin changes characterized by thinning and atrophy. Most intrinsic factors cannot be prevented, but rejuvenative changes can be made with cosmoceutical agents and resurfacing procedures.

Extrinsic factors are preventable environmental influences leading to premature aging of the skin, including ultraviolet (UV) exposure, smoking, chemicals, and gravity. UV exposure is the primary environmental factor, preferentially affecting those with a lighter skin color. The mechanism includes the production of UV-induced oxygen free radicals, which have been shown to invite a cascade of molecular events leading to the production of collagen-degrading enzymes. This creates the characteristic features of photoaging, including rough texture, atrophy, fine and coarse wrinkles, sallow and leathery appearance with dyschromia [1].

In the evaluation of the patient with photoaging, emphasis must be placed on prevention as much as on treatment. Agents available range from cosmoceutical topical agents to filling agents that include resurfacing devices such as chemical peels, ablative resurfacing lasers, and dermabrasion. An initial

---

Facial Resurfacing, 1st edition. Edited by David J. Goldberg. © 2010 Blackwell Publishing.

consultation is performed to determine which of these tools is best for the patient, based on the severity and extent of the condition.

Ablative resurfacing injures the skin in a controlled fashion to a specific depth, encouraging the growth of new and improved skin. These methods include chemical peeling, dermabrasion, and laser resurfacing. Skin resurfacing techniques are divided into superficial, medium-depth, and deep, relating to the level of injury. The deeper procedures are restricted to the face, as other body areas do not have the healing capacity to rejuvenate new skin after such an injury. Care must also be taken with the neck, which may scar with medium-depth or deep injury [2].

The classification system shown in Table 1.1 is useful in categorizing skin resurfacing methods. It is based on the objective data collected by Stegman, who correlated strengths of trichloroacetic acid (TCA) by biopsy to depth of tissue destruction and then new collagen rejuvenation [3]. Thus superficial, medium-depth, and deep resurfacing correlates modalities of peeling, dermabrasion, and laser to common denominators – inflammation and injury.

A useful method of assessing skin-related photoaging is the Monheit–Fulton index (Table 1.2). This system categorizes the visual changes in photoaging skin and quantifies the amount to guide the physician with appropriate therapy. The system combines age-related textural and lesional changes into a numeric system that will predict how aggressive a physician should be in using superficial, medium-depth, and deep resurfacing procedures [4].

Chemical peeling

Chemical peeling remains one of the most popular choices for both patient and physician. In comparison to some of the newer options available, chemical peels have a long-standing safety and efficacy record, are performed with ease, are low in cost, and have a relatively quick recovery time. Various acidic and basic compounds are used to produce a controlled skin injury, and they are classified as superficial, medium-depth, and deep peeling agents according to their level of penetration, destruction, and inflammation (Table 1.1). In general, superficial peels cause epidermal injury and occasionally extend into the papillary dermis, medium-depth peels cause injury through the papillary dermis to the upper reticular dermis, and deep peels cause injury to the mid-reticular dermis [3].

Prior to the application of peeling solutions, the physician must vigorously cleanse the skin surface to remove residual oils, debris, and excess stratum corneum. The face is initially scrubbed with 4″ × 4″ gauze pads containing 0.25% Irgasan (Septisol, Vestal Laboratories, St. Louis, Missouri), then rinsed with water and dried. Because of the defatting and degreasing properties of

Table 1.1 Classification of ablative skin resurfacing methods.

Superficial – very light*
Low-potency formulations of glycolic acid or other alpha-hydroxy acid
10–20% TCA (weight-to-volume formulation)
Jessner's solution (Table 1.3)
Tretinoin
Salicylic acid
Microdermabrasion

Superficial – light*
70% glycolic acid
Jessner's solution
25–35% TCA
Solid CO_2 slush
Microdermabrasion

Medium-depth
88% phenol
35–40% TCA
Jessner's + 35% TCA
70% glycoloic acid + 35% TCA
Solid CO_2 + 35% TCA
Conservative manual dermasanding
Erbium: YAG laser resurfacing
Conservative CO_2 laser resurfacing

Deep
Unoccluded or occluded Baker–Gordon phenol peel
TCA in concentrations > 50%
Wire brush or diamond fraise dermabrasion
Aggressive manual dermasanding
Manual dermasanding or motorized dermabrasion after a medium-depth peel
Aggressive erbium: YAG laser resurfacing
CO_2 laser resurfacing
Combination erbium: YAG/CO_2 laser resurfacing

Although this classification represents an oversimplification, because the actual depth of injury varies somewhat along a continuum for each type of resurfacing procedure, it is helpful when discussing the various options with a patient.
TCA, trichloroacetic acid; YAG, yttrium aluminum garnet.
* Techniques for ablative laser resurfacing of superficial depth have been developed but are probably impractical.

acetone, gauze pads moistened in an acetone preparation are then used to cleanse the skin even further. The importance of cleansing in the peeling procedure cannot be overemphasized. A thorough and evenly distributed cleansing and degreasing of the face ensures uniform penetration of the peeling solution and leads to an even result without skip areas (Fig. 1.1) [5].

Table 1.2 Monheit–Fulton index of photoaging skin.

Texture changes	Points				Score
Wrinkles – dynamic	1	2	3	4	
(% of potential lines)	<25%	<50%	<75%	<100%	
Wrinkles – photoaging	1	2	3	4	
(% of potential lines)	<25%	<50%	<75%	<100%	
Cross-hatched lines – fine lines	1	2	3	4	
(% of potential lines)	<10%	<20%	<40%	<60%	
Sallow color and dyschromia	1	2	3	4	
	Dull	Yellow	Brown	Black	
Leathery appearance	1	2	3	4	
Crinkly (thin & parchment)	1	2	3	4	
Pebbly (deep whitish nodules)	2	4	6	8	
(% of face)	<25%	<50%	<75%	<100%	
Pore # and size	2	4	6	8	
	<25%	<50%	<75%	<100%	

Lesions	Points				Score
Freckles – mottled skin	1	2	3	4	
(# present)	<10	<25	<50	<100	
Lentigenes (dark/irregular)	2	4	6	8	
& SK's (size)	<5 mm	<10 mm	<15 mm	<20 mm	
Telangiectasias – erythema flush	1	2	3	4	
(# present)	<5	<10	<15	>15	
AK's and SK's	2	4	6	8	
(# present)	<5	<10	<15	>15	
Skin cancers	2	4	6	8	
(# present – now or by history)	1 ca	2 ca	3 ca	>4 ca	
Senile comedones	1	2	3	4	
(in cheekbone area)	<5	<10	<20	>20	

Total score					

Corresponding rejuvenation program	
Score	Needs
1–6	Skin care program with tretinoin, glycolic acid peels
7–11	Same plus Jessner's peel; pigmented lesion laser and/or vascular laser
12–16	Same plus medium peel – Jessner's + TCA peel; skin fillers and/or botulinum toxin
17 or more	Above plus laser resurfacing

The effect of a chemical peel is dependent upon the agent used, its concentration, and the techniques employed before and during its application. Each wounding agent used in peels has unique chemical properties and causes a specific pattern of injury to the skin [2]. It is important for the

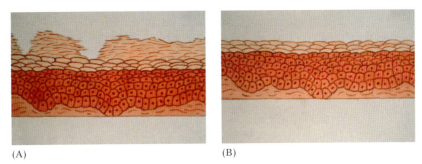

(A)   (B)

Figure 1.1 (A) Irregular surface. (B) Clean, regular surface.

physician using these solutions to be familiar with their cutaneous effects and proper methods of application, to ensure correct depth of injury. This chapter will therefore focus on the specific chemical agents that are actively responsible for producing the various patterns of injury.

Superficial chemical peeling

Superficial chemical peels are indicated in the management of acne and its post-inflammatory erythema, mild photoaging (Glogau I and II), epidermal growths such as lentigines and keratoses, as well as melasma and other pigmentary dyschromias. Multiple peels on a repeated basis are usually necessary to obtain optimal results. The frequency of peels and degree of exposure to the peeling agent may be increased gradually as necessary. Results are enhanced by medical or cosmoceutical therapy. All superficial chemical peels share the advantages of only mild stinging and burning during application, as well as minimal time needed for recovery.

Superficial chemical peels are divided into two varieties – very light and light (Table 1.1). With very light peels, the injury is usually limited to the stratum corneum and only creates exfoliation, but the injury may extend into the stratum granulosum. The agents used for these peels include low-potency formulations of glycolic acid, 10–20% TCA, Jessner's solution (Table 1.3), tretinoin, and salicylic acid. Light peels injure the entire epidermis down to the basal layer, stimulating the regeneration of a fresh new epithelium. Agents used for light peels include 70% glycolic acid, 25–35%

Table 1.3 Jessner's solution (Combe's formula).

Resorcinol	14 g
Salicylic acid	14 g
85% lactic acid	14 g
95% ethanol (QSAD)	100 mL

QSAD, *quantum satis ad dispensum* (quantity sufficient to make the total).

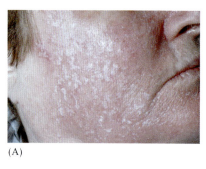
(A)

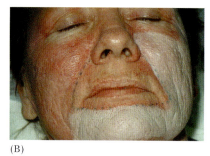
(B)

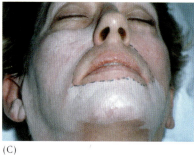
(C)

Figure 1.2 (A) Level I frosting, as found with light chemical peeling: erythema with streaky frosting. (B) Level II: erythema with diffuse white frosting. (C) Level III: solid white enamel frosting.

TCA, Jessner's solution, and solid carbon dioxide slush [6]. During the application of superficial peeling agents, there may be mild stinging followed by a level I frosting, defined as the appearance of erythema and streaky whitening on the surface (Fig. 1.2A, Table 1.4).

Alpha-hydroxy acid (AHA) peeling agents have been used widely in skin rejuvenation programs since the early 1990s. The depth of injury is determined by the specific AHA used, its pH, the concentration of free acid, the volume applied to the skin, and the duration of contact or time the agent is left on the skin before neutralization [7]. In low concentrations (20–30%) AHAs have been shown to decrease the cohesion of corneocytes at the junction of the stratum corneum and the stratum granulosum, while higher concentrations (70%) are associated with complete epidermolysis. Weekly or biweekly applications of 40–70% unbuffered glycolic acid with cotton swabs, a sable brush, or 2″ × 2″ gauze pads have been used most often for acne, mild photoaging, and melasma [7]. The time of application is critical for glycolic acid, as it must be rinsed off with water or neutralized with 5% sodium bicarbonate after 2–4 minutes.

Application of 10–20% TCA with either a saturated 2″ × 2″ gauze pad or sable brush produces erythema and a very light frost within 15–45 seconds. The depth of penetration of the peeling solution is related to the number of coats applied, so deeper penetration and injury can occur with overcoating. Ideally, a level I frosting is obtained with a superficial TCA peel. Protein precipitation results and leads to exfoliation without vesiculation. Concentrations of TCA up to 35% can also be used alone as a superficial peeling agent, but this may create an injury that extends partially into the upper dermis [6].

Jessner's solution is a combination of keratolytic ingredients that has been used for over 100 years in the treatment of inflammatory and comedonal acne as well as hyperkeratotic skin disorders (Table 1.3). Jessner's solution has intense keratolytic activity, initially causing loss of corneocyte cohesion within the stratum corneum and subsequently creating intercellular and intracellular edema within the upper epidermis if application is continued [8]. The mode of application for the Jessner's peel is similar to that of the 10–20% TCA peel. The clinical endpoint of treatment is erythema and blotchy frosting. It is a good repetitive peel for photoaging skin because of its inflammatory effects. The peel can be repeated every 2 weeks.

Salicylic acid, a beta-hydroxy acid that is one of the ingredients in Jessner's solution, can also be used alone in superficial chemical peeling [9]. It is a preferred therapy for comedonal acne as it is lipophilic and concentrates in the pilosebaceous apparatus. It is quite effective as an adjunctive therapy for open and closed comedones and resolving post-acne erythema (Fig. 1.3). It is also a peel of choice for melasma and pigmentary

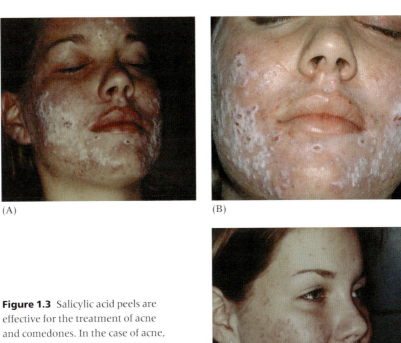

(A)

(B)

Figure 1.3 Salicylic acid peels are effective for the treatment of acne and comedones. In the case of acne, repetitive treatment over six weeks will hasten resolution of the condition. (A) Pre-treatment, active acne. (B) Perifollicular frosting seen with salicylic acid. (C) Six weeks after treatment.

(C)

dyschromia because it has minimal inflammatory action. Used repeatedly, it has the least risk of post-inflammatory hyperpigmentation. For abnormal pigmentation, superficial peeling is combined with skin care and topical retinoids, a bleaching product (including 4–8% hydroquinone), and an adequate sunscreen [10].

Prior to the initial treatment with a superficial peel, both patient and physician must understand the limitations, especially on photoaging, to avoid future disappointment. The effect of repetitive superficial chemical peels never approaches the beneficial effect obtained with a single medium-depth or deep peel. The improvements in photoaged skin following superficial peels are usually subtle, because there is little to no effect on the dermis. Nevertheless, their ease of use and minimal downtime makes these "lunchtime" peels rewarding for patients with realistic expectations.

Medium-depth chemical peeling

Medium-depth chemical peels consist of controlled damage through the epidermis and papillary dermis, with variable extension to the upper reticular dermis. During the next 3 months, postoperatively, there is increased collagen production with expansion of the papillary dermis and the development of a mid-dermal band of thick, elastic-staining fibers [3]. These changes correlate with continued clinical improvement during this time.

For many years, 40–50% TCA was the prototypical medium-depth peeling agent because of its ability to ameliorate fine wrinkles and actinic changes, and to remove pre-neoplasia. TCA as a single agent for medium-depth peeling has fallen out of favor because of the high risk of complications, especially scarring and pigmentary alterations, when used in strengths approaching 50% and higher [11]. Today, most medium-depth chemical peels are performed utilizing 35% TCA in combination with either Jessner's solution, 70% glycolic acid, or solid carbon dioxide (CO_2) as a "priming" agent. These combination peels have been found as effective as 50% TCA alone but with fewer risks. The level of penetration is better controlled with these combination peels, thereby avoiding the scarring seen with higher concentrations of TCA.

Brody developed the use of solid CO_2 to freeze the skin prior to the application of 35% TCA. This causes complete epidermal necrosis and significant dermal edema, thereby allowing deeper penetration of the TCA in selected areas [5]. Monheit then described a combination medium-depth peel in which Jessner's solution is applied, followed by 35% TCA [8]. Similarly, Coleman and Futrell have demonstrated the use of 70% glycolic acid prior to the application of 35% TCA for medium-depth peeling [12]. The Jessner's solution and glycolic acid both appear to effectively weaken the epidermal barrier and allow deeper, more uniform, and more controlled penetration of the 35% TCA.

Current indications for medium-depth chemical peeling include Glogau level II or moderate photoaging, epidermal lesions such as actinic keratoses, pigmentary dyschromias, mild acne scarring, as well as to blend the effects of deeper resurfacing procedures. The most popular of the medium-depth peels for facial rejuvenation is the Jessner's + 35% TCA peel, with other combination peels being utilized less frequently. This peel has been widely accepted because of its broad range of uses, the large number of people in whom it is indicated, its ease of modification according to the situation, and its excellent safety profile. However, it is not a "lunchtime" treatment and should be considered a surgical procedure requiring preoperative consultation and preparation, operative sedation, and aftercare for 1 week or more.

The Jessner's + 35% TCA peel is particularly useful for the improvement of mild to moderate photoaging (Fig. 1.4). It freshens sallow, atrophic skin and softens fine rhytides with minimal risk of textural or pigmentary complications. Collagen remodeling occurs for as long as 3–4 months postoperatively, during which there is continued improvement in texture and rhytides. When used in conjunction with a retinoid, bleaching agent, and sunscreens, a single Jessner's + 35% TCA peel lessens pigmentary dyschromias and lentigines more effectively than repetitive superficial peels (Fig. 1.5). Epidermal growths such as actinic keratoses also respond well to this peel. In fact, the Jessner's + 35% TCA peel has been found as effective as topical 5-fluorouracil chemotherapy in removing both grossly visible and clinically undetectable actinic keratoses, but it has the added advantages of lower morbidity and greater improvement in associated photoaging (Fig. 1.6) [13].

This peel is also useful to blend the effects of other resurfacing procedures with the surrounding skin. Patients who undergo laser resurfacing, deep chemical peeling, or dermabrasion to a localized area such as the periorbital or perioral region often develop a sharp line of demarcation between the treated and untreated skin. This is because the surrounding photoaging skin has significant dyschromia and textural aging. The treated skin may appear hypopigmented (also known as pseudohypopigmentation) in comparison to the untreated skin. A Jessner's + 35% TCA peel performed on the adjacent untreated skin helps to blend the treated area into its surroundings. For example, a patient with advanced photoaging in the periorbital region and moderate photoaging on the remaining face may desire CO_2 laser resurfacing only around her eyes. In this patient, medium-depth chemical peeling of the areas not treated with the laser would improve the photoaging in these regions and avoid a line of demarcation [14]. It is important to note that when used in combination with other resurfacing procedures such as laser resurfacing or dermabrasion, the peel should be

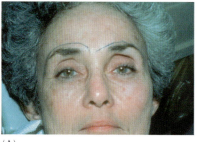

(A)

Monheit Combination Peel

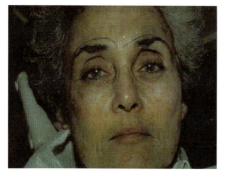

Pre-operative

(B)

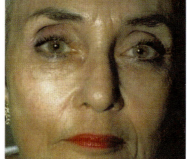

Post-operative

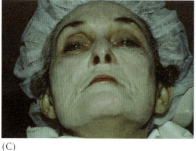

(C)

Figure 1.4 Medium-depth chemical peel used to treat moderate photoaging skin. (A) Preoperative appearance, demonstrating epidermal growths with aging textural changes. (B) Application of 35% TCA directly after Jessner's solution. (C) White enamel frosting (level III) from 35% TCA.

performed first in order to avoid accidental application of the peeling agent onto previously abraded areas of skin (Fig. 1.7).

Using either cotton-tipped applicators or 2″ × 2″ gauze pads, a single, even coat of Jessner's solution is applied first to the forehead, then the cheeks, nose, and chin, and lastly the eyelids. Proper application of Jessner's solution causes minimal discomfort and creates a faint frost within a background of mild erythema (level I). After waiting 1–2 minutes for the Jessner's

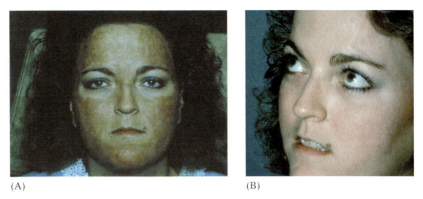

(A)   (B)

Figure 1.5 Post-inflammatory hyperpigmentation unresponsive to topical agents (hydroquinone and tretinoin) and superficial chemical peeling. Full response to medium depth chemical peel and topical agents. (A) Preoperative; (B) six weeks postoperative.

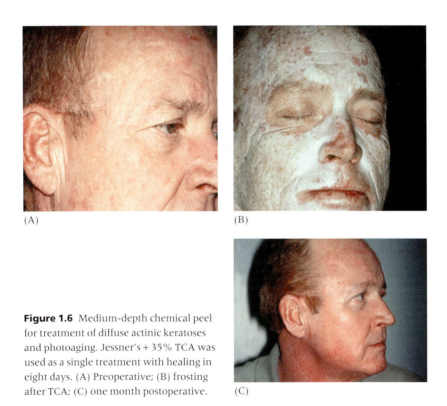

(A)   (B)

Figure 1.6 Medium-depth chemical peel for treatment of diffuse actinic keratoses and photoaging. Jessner's + 35% TCA was used as a single treatment with healing in eight days. (A) Preoperative; (B) frosting after TCA; (C) one month postoperative.

(C)

solution to completely dry, 35% TCA is then applied evenly with one to four cotton-tipped applicators (Fig. 1.8). The effectiveness of this peel is directly dependent upon the depth of penetration of the peeling solutions, and this depth is a function of the adequacy of degreasing and the amount of both solutions applied. The use of cotton swabs, particularly for the

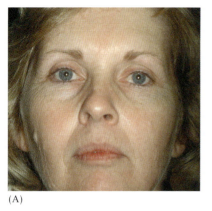

(A)

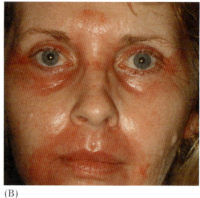

(B)

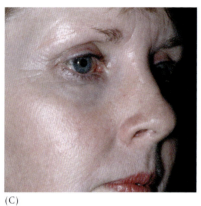

(C)

Figure 1.7 Combination procedure utilizing perioral–periorbital CO_2 laser resurfacing, with Jessner's + 35% TCA peel over remaining face. The peel will blend color and texture of the laser-treated areas. (A) Preoperative: the eyelids and lips need deeper resurfacing than the cheeks, which require only medium-depth injury; (B) four days postoperative: note difference in rate of healing between laser- and peel-treated areas; (C) one year postoperative.

application of TCA, is advantageous because is allows the surgeon to easily vary the amount of solution applied according to the patient's specific needs. The amount of TCA delivered to the skin surface is determined by the number of applicators used, their degree of saturation, the amount of pressure applied to the skin surface, and the duration of their contact with the skin. Four moist cotton-tipped applicators are applied in broad strokes over the forehead and on the medial cheeks. Two mildly soaked cotton-tipped applicators can be used across the lips and chin, and one damp cotton-tipped applicator on the eyelids. The depth of penetration and completion of the peel reaction can be monitored by the level of frosting. A full combination Jessner's + 35% TCA peel should obtain a level II–III frosting. One should never overcoat TCA on a level III frosting, as the injury may be pushed to a level that can cause complications, i.e., pigmentation or scarring.

Anatomic areas of the face are peeled with TCA sequentially from forehead to temple to cheeks, and finally to the lips and eyelids. Careful feathering of the solution into the hairline and around the rim of the jaw and brow conceals the demarcation line between peeled and non-peeled skin. Areas of wrinkled skin are stretched taut with the help of an assistant

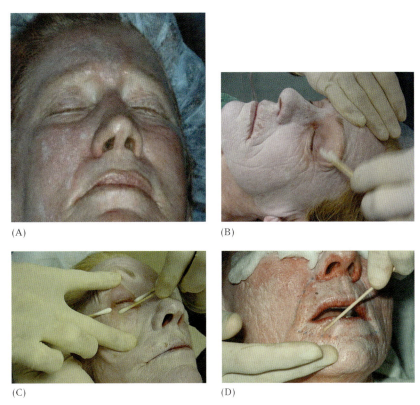

(A)

(B)

(C)

(D)

Figure 1.8 Technical aspects of the Jessner's + 35% TCA peel. (A) Appearance of level I frosting after application of Jessner's solution: erythema with blotchy frosting. (B) 35% TCA applied after Jessner's solution dries with an even application using one to four cotton-tipped applicators: a level III or white enamel frosting is obtained. (C) Eyelids are treated with one cotton-tipped applicator moistened with 35% TCA; a dry applicator is used to absorb tears during eyelid peeling. (D) Lip rhytides are peeled with saturated cotton tip applicators; the wooden shaft is used to rub peel solution further in to the lip rhytides.

to allow even application of the solution into the folds and troughs. This technique is particularly helpful on the skin of the upper and lower lips. For perioral rhytides, TCA is applied with the wood portion of a cotton-tipped applicator and extended onto the vermilion border (Fig. 1.8D).

Eyelid skin must be treated delicately and carefully to avoid over-application and to prevent exposure of the eyes to TCA solution [15]. The patient should be positioned with the head elevated at 30 degrees, and excess peel solution on the cotton tip should be squeezed out so that the applicator is semidry. A single applicator is rolled gently from the periorbital skin onto the upper eyelid skin without going beyond the moveable lid. Another semidry applicator is then rolled onto the lower eyelid skin within 2–3 millimeters of the lid margin while the patient is looking superiorly.

Table 1.4 Grades of frosting with TCA peels.

Grade	Visual finding
I	Erythema with streaky frosting
II	White frosting with visible erythema
III	White enamel frosting – no erythema

Excess peel solution should never be left on the lids, because it can roll into the eyes, and tears should be immediately dried with a cotton-tipped applicator, because they may pull the solution into the eye by capillary action.

The white frost from the TCA application appears on the treated area within 30 seconds to 2 minutes (Fig. 1.4C). This response is representative of keratocoagulation and indicates that the TCA's physiologic reaction is complete. TCA takes longer to frost than phenol preparations, but a shorter period of time than the superficial peeling agents. The desired endpoint in medium-depth peeling is level II–III frosting (Table 1.4). Level II frosting is defined as a white-coated frosting with a background of erythema (Fig. 1.2B).

Level III frosting, which is associated with penetration to the reticular dermis, is a solid white enamel frosting with no background of erythema (Fig. 1.2C). A deeper level III frosting should be restricted only to areas of thick skin and heavy actinic damage. Most medium-depth chemical peels achieve a level II frosting, and this is especially important over the eyelids and areas of sensitive skin. Areas with a greater tendency to form scars, such as the zygomatic arch and the bony prominences of the jawline and chin, should receive no greater than level II frosting.

Before re-treating an area with inadequate frosting, the surgeon should wait at least 3–4 minutes after the application of TCA to ensure that frosting has reached its peak. Each cosmetic unit is then assessed, and areas of incomplete or uneven frosting are carefully re-treated with a thin application of TCA. Additional applications of TCA increase the depth of penetration as well as the risk of complications, so one should apply more solution only to the under-frosted areas.

Although there is an immediate burning sensation as the peel solution is applied, the discomfort begins to subside as frosting occurs and resolves fully by the time of discharge. This peel can be performed with light sedation, such as:
- diazepam 10 mg orally
- meperidine 50 mg intramuscularly
- hydroxyzine 25 mg intramuscularly

After cooling the skin with saline, the patient will remain comfortable throughout the postoperative period. Cool saline compresses offer symptomatic relief at the conclusion of the peel. Unlike the compresses in glycolic acid peels, the saline following a TCA peel simply provides relief and does not "neutralize" the acid.

Deep chemical peeling

Patients with more extreme skin photoaging may require deep chemical peeling, motorized dermabrasion, or laser resurfacing to improve their greater degree of skin damage. As discussed with medium-depth peels, deep chemical peeling leads to production of new collagen and ground substance down to a level in proportion to the depth of the peel. The peeling agent of choice is the Baker–Gordon phenol peel.

The Baker–Gordon peel utilizes phenol in a formulation that permits deep penetration into the dermis, deeper than full-strength phenol [16]. The Baker–Gordon formula consists of Septisol (Vestal Laboratories, St. Louis, MO), croton oil, and tap water added to a solution of phenol, reducing its concentration to 50% or 55% (Table 1.5). The mixture of ingredients is freshly prepared and must be stirred vigorously prior to application due to its poor miscibility. The liquid soap, Septisol, is a surfactant that reduces skin tension, allowing a more even penetration. Croton oil is a vesicant epidermolytic agent that enhances phenol absorption. Recent investigations into the effects of this peel using varying concentrations of both phenol and croton oil have suggested that the procedure's efficacy is related more to the amount of croton oil than to the phenol [17,18].

There are two main variations in deep chemical peeling with the Baker–Gordon phenol formula: occluded and unoccluded. Occlusion of the peeling solution with tape is thought to increase its penetration and extend the injury into the mid-reticular dermis. This technique is particularly helpful for deeply lined, "weather-beaten" faces but should be utilized only by experienced surgeons because of the higher risk of complications [19]. The unoccluded technique as modified by McCollough involves a more vigorous cleansing of the skin and the application of more peel solution [20]. This may enhance the efficacy of the solution, but without penetration as

Table 1.5 The Baker–Gordon formula.

88% liquid phenol, USP	3 mL
Tap water	2 mL
Septisol liquid soap	8 drops
Croton oil	3 drops

USP, United States Pharmacopeia.

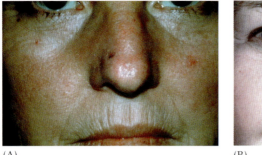
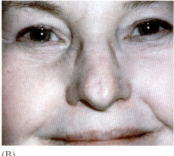

(A)   (B)

Figure 1.9 Advanced photoaging of perioral rhytides treated with Baker–Gordon phenol peel. (A) Preoperative appearance, demonstrating perioral rhagades, textural and pigmentary changes with epidermal growths. (B) Postoperative, two years later: note that the phenol peel maintains correction for many years.

deep as in an occluded peel. In the hands of a skilled and knowledgeable surgeon, both methods are safe and reliable in rejuvenating advanced to severe photoaged skin. Deep chemical peeling can significantly improve or even eliminate deep furrows as well as other textural and pigmentary irregularities associated with severe photoaging (Fig. 1.9). A remarkable degree of improvement is the expected result of deep chemical peeling when performed properly on carefully selected patients.

The patient undergoing deep chemical peeling must understand and be willing to accept the significant risk of complications and the increased degree of morbidity. The most notable complications include scarring, textural changes such as "alabaster skin" or "plastic skin," and pigmentary disturbances. It is not uncommon for patients to experience postoperative erythema that can take many months to resolve and may be followed by variable hypopigmentation (Fig. 1.10). Male patients and patients with darker complexions are less favorable candidates for deep chemical peeling, as the hypopigmentation is less easily camouflaged. Since phenol is cardiotoxic, preoperative evaluation includes a complete blood count, liver function tests, serum urea nitrogen and creatinine and electrolyte determinations, and a baseline electrocardiogram. Any patient who has a history

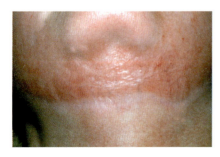

Figure 1.10 Complications from Baker–Gordon phenol peel with prolonged non-healing, resulting in hypopigmentation and marbled scarring.

of cardiac arrhythmias or who is taking a medication known to precipitate arrhythmias should not undergo a full-face Baker–Gordon phenol peel. Patients with a history of hepatic or renal disease are also poor candidates.

Compared with medium-depth and superficial peeling, the Baker–Gordon phenol peel is a time-consuming procedure, and it must be performed only in a properly equipped facility. The required waiting period after the treatment of each cosmetic unit limits the rate of cutaneous absorption, thereby preventing the serum levels of phenol from reaching a dangerous peak during the procedure. Intravenous hydration with a liter of lactated Ringer's solution before the procedure and another liter during the peel also promotes phenol excretion and prevents toxicity. Continuous electrocardiography, pulse oximetry, and blood pressure monitoring are mandatory during the entire perioperative period. Any abnormalities, such as a premature ventricular contraction (PVC) or premature atrial contraction (PAC), necessitate abrupt stoppage of the procedure and careful evaluation for toxicity [21]. Oxygen is supplemented throughout the procedure, as some physicians feel that it has a protective effect against cardiac arrhythmias.

After thorough cleansing and degreasing of the skin, the chemical agent is applied sequentially to six aesthetic units: forehead, perioral region, right cheek, left cheek, nose, and periorbital region. There is a 15-minute interval between the treatment of each cosmetic area, allowing 60–90 minutes for the entire procedure. Cotton-tipped applicators are used with a technique similar to that described for the medium-depth Jessner's + 35% TCA peel, although less solution is used because frosting occurs very rapidly (Fig. 1.11). Occlusion of the peel can be accomplished with strips of waterproof zinc oxide tape (e.g., half-inch Curity tape) to each cosmetic unit just after the phenol is applied. Care is exercised to extend the peel slightly beyond the mandibular rim, to conceal the demarcation between treated and untreated skin. The last aesthetic unit, the periorbital skin, is treated cautiously and conservatively to avoid over-penetration, which can lead to ectropion or scarring. It is important to remember that diluting a phenol compound with water may increase its penetration, so mineral oil rather than water should be used to flush the eyes if contact occurs.

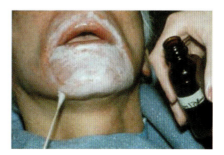

Figure 1.11 Rapid frosting from small amounts of Baker's phenol solution applied with cotton-tipped applicators.

Application of the peeling agent creates an immediate burning sensation, which lasts for 15–20 seconds, subsides for 20 minutes, and then returns for the next 6–8 hours. Ice packs may be applied as necessary for patient comfort. Narcotics are usually prescribed upon discharge for adequate pain control. Systemic steroids are also administered by some surgeons to lessen the inflammatory response. For untaped peels, petrolatum is applied and a biosynthetic dressing can be used for the first 24 hours.

Conclusion

There are multiple instruments now available for resurfacing and retexturing photodamaged and aging skin. Although new fractional non-ablative and ablative lasers are appealing because of skin contraction and less downtime, non-ablative lasers can produce results very similar to light chemical peels, with minimal downtime. With these choices available, it behooves the cosmetic physician to be familiar with chemical peeling as a major tool in the practice. The medium-depth peel especially is a reliable procedure that is efficacious and safe for most patients. The results are individualized to each patient's needs, though the physician needs the training and experience to perform the procedure correctly.

References

1 Leyden JJ. Photodamage: an overview. *Skin Allergy News* 2003 (supplement, July); 3–4.
2 Monheit GD, Chastain MA. Chemical peels. *Facial Plast Surg Clin North Am* 2001; **9**: 239–55.
3 Stegman SJ. A comparative histologic study of the effects of three peeling agents and dermabrasion on normal and sundamaged skin. *Aesthetic Plast Surg* 1982; **6**: 123–35.
4 Monheit GD. Presentations at the American Academy of Dermatology in New Orleans, March 25, 1999.
5 Monheit GD. Skin preparation: an essential step before chemical peeling or laser resurfacing. *Cosmet Dermatol* 1996; **9** (9): 13–14.
6 Brody HJ. *Chemical Peeling*. St. Louis, MO: Mosby Year Book, 1992, pp. 59–60.
7 Moy LS, Murad H, Moy RL. Glycolic acid peels for the treatment of wrinkles and photoaging. *J Dermatol Surg Oncol* 1993; **19**: 243–6.
8 Monheit GD. The Jessner's + TCA peel: a medium depth chemical peel. *J Dermatol Surg Oncol* 1989; **15**: 945–50.
9 Kligman D, Kligman AM. Salicylic acid peels for the treatment of photoaging. *Dermatol Surg* 1998; **24**: 325–8.
10 Monheit GD. Chemical peeling for pigmentary dyschromias. *Cosmet Dermatol* 1995; **8** (5): 10–15.
11 Brody HJ, Hailey CW. Medium-depth chemical peeling of the skin: a variation of superficial chemosurgery. *J Dermatol Surg Oncol* 1986; **12**: 1268–75.

12 Coleman WP, Futrell JM. The glycolic acid trichloroacetic acid peel. *J Dermatol Surg Oncol* 1994; 20: 76–80.

13 Witheiler DD, Lawrence N, Cox SE, Cruz C, Cockerell CJ, Freemen RG. Long-term efficacy and safety of Jessner's solution and 35% trichloroacetic acid vs 5% fluorouracil in the treatment of widespread facial actinic keratoses. *Dermatol Surg* 1997; **23**: 191–6.

14 Monheit GD. The Jessner's–TCA peel. *Facial Plast Surg Clin North Am* 1994; **2**: 21–7.

15 Morrow DM. Chemical peeling of eyelids and periorbital area. *J Dermatol Surg Oncol* 1992; **18**: 102–10.

16 Baker TS, Gordon HL. Chemical Face Peeling. In: *Surgical Rejuvenation of the Face*. St. Louis, MO: Mosby Year Book, 1986, pp. 230–2.

17 Hetter GP. An examination of the phenol-croton oil peel. Part I. Dissecting the formula. *Plast Reconstr Surg* 2000; **105**: 227–39; discussion 249–51.

18 Hetter GP. An examination of the phenol-croton oil peel. Part IV. Face peel results with different concentrations of phenol and croton oil. *Plast Reconstr Surg* 2000; **105**: 1061–83; discussion 1084–7.

19 Alt T. Occluded Baker–Gordon chemical peel: review and update. *J Dermatol Surg Oncol* 1989; **15**: 980–93.

20 McCollough EG, Langsdon PR. Chemical peeling with phenol. In: Roenigk H, Roenigk R, eds., *Dermatologic Surgery: Principles and Practice*. New York, NY: Marcel Dekker, 1989, pp. 997–1016.

21 Beeson WH. The importance of cardiac monitoring in superficial and deep chemical peeling. *J Dermatol Surg Oncol* 1987; **13**: 949–50.

CHAPTER 2

Non-Ablative Resurfacing

Alexander L. Berlin[1,2] and David J. Goldberg[3]

[1] Edward E. Rotan, Jr., M.D., P.A., Arlington and Sugar Land, TX, USA
[2] New Jersey Medical School, Newark, NY, USA
[3] Mount Sinai School of Medicine, New York, NY, USA

Key points

- Non-ablative resurfacing became popular as a response to the problems associated with older ablative devices
- Intense pulsed light sources and mid-infrared lasers are the most commonly used non-ablative devices
- Non-ablative devices are associated with rare side effects
- Non-ablative devices, later replaced by fractional non-ablative devices, do not produce the degree of improvement seen with fractional ablative lasers

---

Introduction

With the proven success of older non-fractional ablative resurfacing technologies, the search for non-invasive rejuvenation got under way. Nicknamed "lunchtime rejuvenation," non-ablative resurfacing aims to improve the visible signs of photoaging without visible damage to the epidermis and, consequently, minimal to no downtime. Also known as subsurface remodeling, non-ablative photorejuvenation has thus become an acceptable treatment modality for a large number of patients who cannot or are not willing to endure a prolonged downtime or to undergo expensive and potentially risky surgical corrective procedures. Later replaced by fractional non-ablative lasers and, most recently, by today's popular fractional ablative devices, non-ablative resurfacing is still in use today. Although typically only subtle clinical improvement is achieved, patients with mild to moderate photoaging and realistic expectations are good candidates for this procedure.

The devices that will be discussed in this chapter – including intense pulsed light (IPL) sources and mid-infrared lasers – have been found not only to improve an individual component of photoaged skin, such as pigmented or vascular lesions, but also to contribute to dermal remodeling following full-facial treatment.

Facial Resurfacing, 1st edition. Edited by David J. Goldberg. © 2010 Blackwell Publishing.

Laser–tissue interactions and subsurface remodeling

Clinical improvement following ablative resurfacing has been found to be more closely related to the residual thermal damage, or thermal diffusion, and subsequent collagen denaturation and fibroplasia than to the optical penetration depth by the laser beam [1,2]. Similarly, although not completely elucidated, the mechanism of action of most non-ablative resurfacing devices is thought to involve collagen denaturation.

Collagens I and III, which belong to the fibril-forming family of collagens, contribute significantly to the dermal extracellular matrix network. The collagen molecule is a right-handed helix with three polypeptide chains, known as alpha-chains, held together by hydrogen bonds between the hydroxyl groups of the hydroxyproline residues [3]. These relatively weak hydrogen bonds break upon heating, leading to a random-coil configuration of the alpha-chains and subsequent shortening and thickening of the fibrils [4,5].

Dermal heating may be accomplished through bulk heating of the water content or the propagation of heat from dermal structures, such as the blood vessels. However, unlike that seen in ablative resurfacing, dermal remodeling in non-ablative rejuvenation occurs in an upside-down manner. This is achieved via dermal heating with concomitant epidermal cooling. Because of the resultant epidermal sparing, the subsequent biological effect is sometimes referred to as "subsurface remodeling." In the process, the ensuing wound-healing response eventuates in the proliferation and the activation of dermal fibroblasts, which, in turn, begin to lay down new collagen fibers [6,7].

Additional biological processes may contribute to the clinical improvement following non-ablative resurfacing and will need to be uncovered in future studies.

Patient selection and pre-procedural care

Considering the somewhat milder improvement obtained with the help of non-ablative technologies, proper patient selection is crucial to the success of the procedure. The best candidates for the procedure are between 35 and 55 years of age with mildly to moderately photodamaged facial skin, manifesting as early rhytides, increased skin fragility, poor elasticity, coarse texture, and increased pore size. Younger patients may have few, if any, clinically noticeable cutaneous irregularities, making any improvement difficult to discern. On the other hand, older patients are more likely to have deeper rhytides and more severe textural alterations, and may therefore not be adequately satisfied with the outcome of the procedure. For the latter group, ablative resurfacing using deeper chemical peels or laser-based technologies, as described in other chapters, may be better therapeutic options. In all cases, high-quality multiple-angle photographs should be obtained prior to treatment in order to document subsequent improvement, as subtle gradual changes may not be readily apparent to the patient.

Depending on the selected non-ablative rejuvenating technology, the patient's skin tone may be an important consideration. Thus, IPL sources and certain mid-infrared lasers may require specific modifications of treatment parameters in order to avoid potential complications. This stems from the fact that epidermal melanin may act as a competing chromophore in the skin. Absorption by melanin progressively decreases with increasing wavelengths and becomes nearly negligible in the infrared portion of the electromagnetic spectrum. Thus, longer wavelengths may be safer in patients with darker skin tones or in the presence of a suntan; nonetheless, excessive fluences and prolonged cryogen exposure may still contribute to dyschromia in such individuals. These considerations will be further discussed with the specific corresponding technologies.

Photosensitivity to the emitted wavelengths and active inflammatory or infectious cutaneous disease in the proposed treatment area are contraindications to non-ablative rejuvenation. The safety of these devices in pregnant or lactating females has not been adequately studied; in addition, their use in this population is best avoided because of a greater propensity towards hyperpigmentation [8]. Finally, a history of excessive or keloidal scarring should be sought prior to treatment.

Although a controversial topic, oral isotretinoin intake within 6 months of ablative, aggressive resurfacing techniques, such as dermabrasion, may lead to a higher risk of delayed wound healing and keloidal scarring [9–11]. It is unclear, however, whether the same contraindication applies to non-ablative technologies, as there have been no published reports of such a complication following these less aggressive procedures. In addition, prior injection of botulinum neurotoxin A or intradermal fillers is not a contraindication to non-ablative resurfacing, as the procedure does not inactivate or cause migration of the product [12,13].

Although the procedures are generally well tolerated, topical anesthetic agents may be utilized with higher fluences or based on patient preferences. Makeup should be removed prior to treatment to prevent light absorption and subsequent epidermal burn. Finally, eye protection in the form of goggles should be provided to the patient and all treating and assisting personnel.

Intense pulsed light sources

The versatility of IPL devices allows them to be used for various clinical indications, such as the treatment of pigmented and vascular lesions (Figs. 2.1–2.3). While such lesions form part of the changes frequently

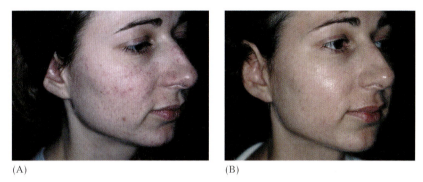

(A)   (B)

Figure 2.1 Intense pulsed light treatment: (A) before treatment; (B) after treatment.

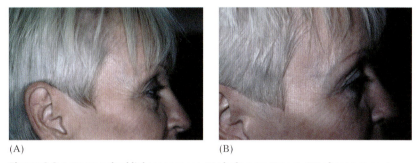

(A)   (B)

Figure 2.2 Intense pulsed light treatment: (A) before treatment; (B) after treatment.

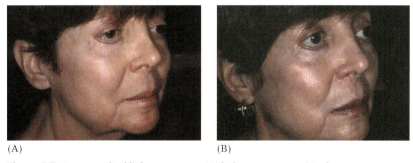

(A)   (B)

Figure 2.3 Intense pulsed light treatment: (A) before treatment; (B) after treatment.

Table 2.1 Commonly used intense pulsed light (IPL) sources.

Name	Manufacturer	Spectral output (nm)
Lumenis One	Lumenis	515–1200
IPL Quantum	Lumenis	560–1200
StarLux 300 and 500	Palomar	
• LuxG handpiece		500–670 & 870–1200
• LuxV handpiece		400–700 & 870–1200
• LuxY handpiece		525–1200
Clareon with SR handpiece	Novalis Medical	550–1200
PhotoLight and Photosilk Plus	Cynosure	400–1200
BBL	Sciton	420–1400

noted in photoaged skin, IPL devices are able to effect dermal remodeling, thereby achieving overall photorejuvenation. In the original study of this device for full-face rejuvenation, a significant clinical improvement in rhytides, skin texture, and pore size was documented, in addition to that in the epidermal dyspigmentation and telangiectasias [14]. Subsequent clinical studies confirmed these findings [15,16]. Furthermore, histological evidence of fibroblast stimulation, neocollagenesis, and subsequent dermal remodeling for up to 6 months following the treatment has also been documented [17,18]. Additional microscopic effects of IPL non-ablative resurfacing include increased epidermal thickness, formation of new rete ridges, decreased horny plugs, and decreased solar elastosis [19].

Because of a wide variation in the currently available IPL sources (Table 2.1) – including differences in the spectral output and filters, pulse shape and duration, spot size, and the generated fluences – direct comparison of clinical outcomes and, consequently, determination of optimal settings is somewhat difficult. Nonetheless, relevant and important generalizations can be made to guide the practitioner. In addition, most manufacturers have developed specific treatment recommendations, frequently included as preprogrammed parameters in user-friendly menus. For older devices or those without incorporated presets, consulting a user manual or communicating directly with the manufacturer is recommended.

Unlike lasers, IPL devices are polychromatic sources of light. As previously mentioned, their spectral outputs may vary, but usually fall within the 400–1400 nm range. While the actual spectral output of each device is proprietary, a greater proportion of the emitted light is typically in the shorter wavelengths. On the other hand, most devices emit little energy beyond 1000 nm. Thus the effective output may be controlled with cutoff filters in order to achieve target selectivity, as dictated by the principle of selective photothermolysis [20]. Most devices feature either interchangeable high-pass filters or separate handpieces that block out most light emission below the rated wavelength (Table 2.1).

The choice of a proper filter depends on several factors, including the patient's skin type, the presence of a suntan, and the specific aspects of photoaging being addressed in a given patient. Lower wavelengths, such as those in the 515–590 nm range, are especially effective in the treatment of telangiectasias; however, purpura may be encountered at the lower end of this range. The tissue target in light-based treatment of epidermal pigmented lesions and dyschromia is melanin; as mentioned previously, its absorption gradually decreases over the visible light spectrum. Therefore, these lower wavelengths may be used to concurrently treat increased vascularity and pigmentation. On the other hand, filters in the 600–700 nm range may allow for selective elimination of epidermal dyschromia with a reduced incidence of erythema or purpura. Such wavelengths are also safer in individuals with a darker complexion or those with a suntan, in whom post-inflammatory hyperpigmentation or hypopigmented footprints, respectively, may otherwise be encountered post-treatment. Importantly, both the lower- and the higher-range wavelengths have been shown to be effective in the improvement of the other aspects of photoaged skin, including coarse texture, increased pore size, and fine rhytides [14,21].

IPL devices are long-pulsed systems. Thus, rather than being continuous, IPL emission is pulsatile in nature. The characteristics of such emission include pulse shape, pulse duration, and pulse stacking. Pulse shape depends on the specific system and cannot be adjusted. Thus, in certain systems, full fluence is delivered from the start of the emission, giving the pulse a square shape, whereas others achieve full fluence only after a delay, resulting in a more trapezoid pulse shape. Pulse duration, or pulse width, is usually adjustable and is selected based on the thermal relaxation time (TRT) of the specific lesion being treated, as explained by the theory of selective photothermolysis [20]. TRT is directly proportional to the square of the size of the object; thus, smaller targets, such as minute telangiectasias, require relatively short pulse durations. On the other hand, longer exposure allows for greater heat propagation, dermal heating and collagen denaturation, and, ultimately, greater photorejuvenation. Longer pulse durations are also safer in darker individuals or those with a suntan, as the epidermal melanin is allowed sufficient time to dissipate heat and to cool down. Additionally, longer pulse durations may be subdivided in some systems into two or more stacked pulses with a preset or variable inter-pulse delay. Such delay may also allow for epidermal cooling and may be safer in patients with skin types IV and V [22].

A distinguishing feature of many of the modern IPL devices is their large spot size, in some instances reaching over 8 cm^2 in surface area. A large spot size has two advantages. First, the treatment of large surfaces, such as full face, is very rapid. Second, as with lasers, greater spots result in a smaller percentage of the light beam being scattered by dermal collagen and, consequently, greater beam penetration. Some devices feature interchangeable spot sizes for smaller surfaces. Based on the above explanation, fluence needs to be increased when a smaller spot size is selected, and decreased with the larger spots.

As could be deduced from the large variability in the above-mentioned parameters, fluences cannot be directly compared across the different systems, sometimes even by the same manufacturer. This problem is further compounded by varying calibration techniques employed by the manufacturers [23]. The practitioner is advised to use the included presets, if available, or to consult the user manual or the manufacturer for the recommended initial fluence, based on the patient's skin type and the other settings as delineated above.

Finally, concurrent epidermal cooling serves to provide further epidermal protection, as well as topical anesthesia. In most systems, this is accomplished with the help of a chilled sapphire or quartz tip; few utilize cryogen spray cooling. Additional cooling is afforded by a chilled ultrasound gel applied to the treatment area, which also serves to reduce light refraction by the air. Although important for all patients, epidermal cooling is critical in those with the darker skin tones, and should be tested immediately prior to treatment.

Several non-ablative resurfacing sessions – typically 3–6 – are required to achieve an impressive and long-lasting improvement in the signs of photoaging using an IPL device [14,15]. These may be performed every 2–4 weeks; this interval may be lengthened in patients with darker skin tones to allow for resolution of any post-inflammatory hyperpigmentation.

Adverse effects following non-ablative resurfacing with IPL devices are generally mild and short-lived. Erythema and edema are expected in most cases, but mostly resolve in 1–2 days; these may be accompanied by a burning or stinging sensation or pain. Furthermore, the duration of erythema may be reduced by post-procedural exposure to light-emitting diode (LED) devices [24]. As was previously mentioned, purpura may also occur, especially with the shorter wavelengths, but tends to last only 2–5 days, as opposed to the 5–14 days commonly seen in association with a pulsed dye laser [25]. Blistering, which may subsequently result in erosions, is seen in up to 10% of the treated patients but usually resolves without sequelae [26]. Patients should therefore be warned not to manipulate any blisters, if any appear following treatment.

Transient discoloration following IPL photorejuvenation may be an expected consequence or a potential complication of treatment. Thus, epidermal pigmented lesions, such as lentigines or ephelides, initially become darker, followed by eventual desquamation within 3–7 days. Since this is an expected occurrence, patients should be appropriately forewarned to prevent unnecessary distress. More prolonged dyschromia, including hypo- and hyperpigmentation, may be seen in up to 15% of patients, especially those with darker skin tones, a suntan, or melasma within the treatment area [27]. Such dyschromia usually lasts less than 2 months, and its incidence may be reduced – though likely not entirely eliminated – by following the above-mentioned guidelines regarding various device settings.

Finally, because of its absorption of light throughout the visible portion of the electromagnetic spectrum, melanin contained within hair shafts and follicles represents an important consideration in IPL-mediated photorejuvenation. The device aperture must be kept at least 2 mm away from the eyebrows to prevent epilation. Likewise, male patients must be warned about a potential for temporary hair loss if the beard or the mustache area is treated.

Mid-infrared lasers

Mid-infrared wavelengths have a long track record of improving all aspects of photoaged skin (Figs. 2.4–2.9). It should not come as a surprise, therefore, that the original fractional non-ablative devices, were also based on these wavelengths. Traditional, non-fractionated mid-infrared lasers frequently utilized for non-ablative facial photorejuvenation include 1319/1320 nm neodymium:yttrium–aluminum–garnet (Nd:YAG) lasers, a 1450 nm diode laser, and a 1540 nm ytterbium–erbium:phosphate glass laser, also known as an erbium:glass (Er:glass) laser (Table 2.2).

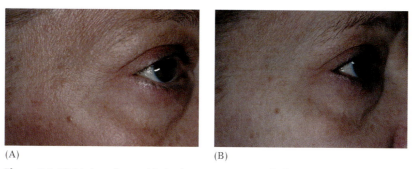

(A)   (B)

Figure 2.4 Mid-infrared non-ablative laser treatment: (A) before treatment; (B) after treatment.

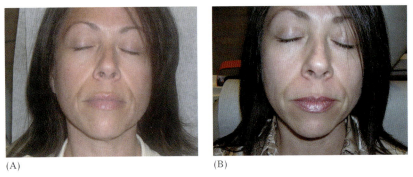

(A)   (B)

Figure 2.5 Mid-infrared non-ablative laser treatment: (A) before treatment;
(B) after treatment.

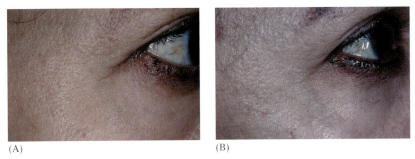

(A)   (B)

Figure 2.6 Mid-infrared non-ablative laser treatment: (A) before treatment;
(B) after treatment.

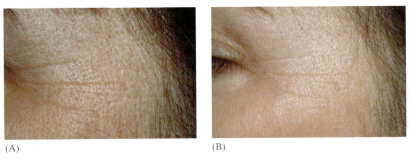

(A)   (B)

Figure 2.7 Mid-infrared non-ablative laser treatment: (A) before treatment;
(B) after treatment.

Light in the mid-infrared portion of the electromagnetic spectrum is preferentially absorbed by water. In fact, little absorption by oxyhemoglobin
occurs beyond 1200 nm, while most of absorption by melanin is within the
visible and near-infrared portions of the spectrum. Thus, these laser systems
are safe in all skin types, as long as proper exposure and cooling settings are
employed, as described below. In the case of the three commonly utilized

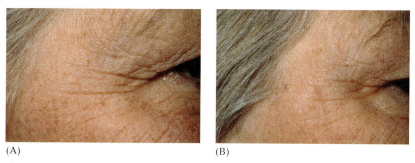

(A)   (B)

Figure 2.8 Mid-infrared non-ablative laser treatment: (A) before treatment;
(B) after treatment.

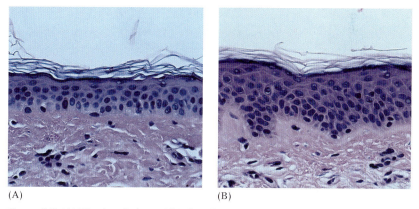

(A)   (B)

Figure 2.9 (A) Histology before mid-infrared non-ablative laser treatment;
(B) histologic changes after mid-infrared non-ablative laser treatment: note thickened
dermis with new collagen formation.

Table 2.2 Commonly used mid-infrared lasers.

Name	Manufacturer	Wavelength (nm)
CoolTouch CT3	CoolTouch	1320
ThermaScan	Sciton	1319
SmoothBeam	Candela	1450
Aramis	Quantel Medical	1540

wavelengths, water has the lowest absorption coefficient at 1320 nm,
allowing for a slightly greater optical penetration depth [28]. However,
dermal scatter decreases as the wavelength of light increases. Thus, the
mid-infrared lasers likely have very comparable clinical efficacy, although

direct comparisons utilizing the latest models of each laser system in the improvement of photoaged skin are lacking.

Most of the clinical effect achieved by these lasers is thought to arise from dermal water heating with subsequent collagen denaturation and remodeling. In fact, several histological analyses have confirmed immediate post-exposure shortening and thickening of the collagen fibrils, followed by fibroblast proliferation and deposition of new collagen types I and III [6,7,29] (Fig. 2.9). Subsurface remodeling is then thought to be responsible for the clinical improvement in skin texture, tone, and fine rhytides that accompanies these microscopic changes [6,7,30]. It should, however, be noted that fibroblast activation and subsequent collagen remodeling is a delayed process; thus, full clinical impact may not always be apparent for up to 4–6 months following a series of treatments, as delineated below [31].

In addition, some studies have noted vascular damage in the papillary dermis and basal layer edema following irradiation with a mid-infrared laser. These changes were accompanied by a neutrophilic inflammatory infiltrate [32]. It has therefore been proposed that additional factors, possibly involving various cytokines and chemokines, may be involved in dermal remodeling. In fact, a statistically significant increase in pro-inflammatory cytokines IL-1β and TNF-α, as well as in matrix metalloproteinases 1 and 9 (MMP-1 and MMP-9), has been demonstrated [33]. The relative contribution of these factors to the process of neocollagenesis and collagen remodeling remains unclear at this time.

The above-mentioned basal-layer edema, accompanied by epidermal spongiosis, is an important consideration, as normally subclinical damage to the epidermis may result in clinically evident blistering if proper epidermal protection in the form of epidermal cooling is not provided. This epidermal damage may result from water absorption within the epidermis, backscatter with subepidermal concentration of heat, or heat propagation from the upper dermis. Case in point, the early 1320 nm laser systems featuring only pre-pulse epidermal cooling resulted in a higher incidence of scarring [34]. Thus, all current mid-infrared lasers feature pre-, intra-, and post-exposure epidermal cooling, accomplished with either multiple spurts of cryogen spray or continuous contact cooling with a chilled sapphire tip (Table 2.2). Care must be taken, however, as excessive exposure to cryogen may cause frostbite-type epidermal injury with potential subsequent dyschromia and atrophic scarring, especially in individuals with darker skin tones.

The 1320 nm Nd:YAG laser features a fixed 50 ms pulse duration consisting of six stacked pulses and a fixed 10 mm spot size. Furthermore, the handpiece is equipped with a thermal sensor that is brought into contact with the skin during emission. A measured epidermal temperature of 40–45 °C correlates well with dermal heating to approximately 70 °C and the resulting collagen denaturation. On the other hand, temperatures above 48 °C have been found to result in an excessive risk of epidermal injury [32]. Thus, the initial fluence is usually set to 12–18 J/cm² and a test firing is performed. Fluence is then adjusted to achieve the desired epidermal temperature. Finally, cryogen spray is released in three spurts to achieve pre-, intra-, and post-exposure cooling. The duration of each of the three spurts is measured in milliseconds and is adjustable. As per the above discussion, this duration should be reduced in darkly complexioned patients to prevent cold injury [34].

In addition to its variable pulse duration and spot size, a separate commercially available 1319 nm Nd:YAG laser (Table 2.2) also features continuous contact cooling with a chilled sapphire tip, which may be associated with less discomfort and lower incidence of cold injury due to the cryogen. Exposures may be delivered singly or scanned in a non-sequential pattern to prevent adjacent epidermal overheating.

The 1450 nm diode laser has a fixed total pulse duration of 210 ms, consisting of four stacked pulses and spot sizes of 4 and 6 mm. For the purpose of photorejuvenation, fluence is usually set between 9 and 14 J/cm², but may be adjusted depending on patient tolerance and the perceived clinical efficacy. Finally, epidermal protection is afforded by five cryogen spurts delivered pre-, intra-, and post-exposure. As with the 1320 nm laser, cryogen exposure should be limited in patients with darker skin tones to prevent injury and subsequent dyschromia or scarring.

Finally, the 1540 nm Er:glass laser features a 4 mm spot size and has a pulse duration of 3 ms in a single-pulse, or normal, mode, with up to three pulses delivered per second in a pulse-train mode. For the purpose of photorejuvenation, the initial fluence is typically set to 8–10 J/cm² per pulse in the single-pulse mode. When the pulse-train mode is selected, the cumulative fluence should be limited to 60 J/cm² to avoid epidermal damage [35–37]. Instead of cryogen spray, this device utilizes continuous contact cooling with a sapphire tip, which may be associated with less intra-treatment patient discomfort.

As with the IPL devices, several treatment sessions – typically between three and six – are required for significant long-term clinical improvement in the various aspects of photoaged facial skin [38–40]. Treatments may be undertaken every 2–4 weeks, allowing sufficient time for the complete resolution of any residual erythema. As mentioned previously, the full impact of this non-ablative resurfacing may not be apparent until 4–6 months following the procedure.

Adverse effects are typically mild following treatment with mid-infrared lasers. Transient mild to moderate pain may be experienced during and immediately following the procedure; however, topical anesthesia is unnecessary in most cases. Mild erythema and edema are short-lasting and typically resolve within 1–3 days [41]. Finally, dyschromia and blistering are uncommon with these lasers, but usually resolve without scarring [39,40]. These may occur in the setting of excessive fluences or cryogen exposure.

Fractional non-ablative infrared lasers

In 2004 Manstein *et al.* introduced the concept of fractional non-ablative photothermolysis using an erbium-doped fiber laser (Fraxel, Solta Medical Inc., Hayward, CA) in an attempt to deliver better results than were seen with traditional non-ablative lasers, without the associated risks and lengthy recovery period seen with their ablative counterparts (Fig. 2.10). Whereas traditional laser resurfacing removes the entire top layer of the skin surface, creating a visible wound and loss of the skin's protective function, fractional laser resurfacing treats a small "fraction" of the skin at each session. This also differs from other non-ablative lasers, which require epidermal cooling while they heat the dermis and hence produce no resurfacing effect. Intact, undamaged skin around each treated area theoretically acts as a barrier to infection and a reservoir for rapid healing through migration of surrounding epidermal cells and division of transient amplifying cells from the basal layer [42].

The Fraxel laser was the first laser that utilized fractional technology at a wavelength of 1550 nm to coagulate the epidermis and dermis. Subsequently, a number of other lasers and light-based devices have utilized fractional technology (Table 2.3).

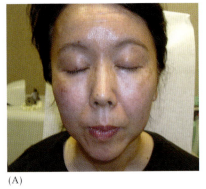 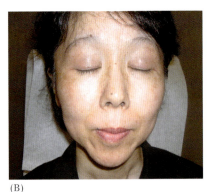

(A)   (B)

Figure 2.10 Fractional non-ablative laser treatment: (A) photodamage and melasma before treatment; (B) improvement after treatment.

Table 2.3 Commonly used fractional non-ablative devices.

Name	Manufacturer	Wavelength (nm)
Fraxel SR	Solta Medical	1550
StarLux 300 and 500	Palomar	
• Lux1540 Fractional handpiece		1540
• Lux1440 Fractional handpiece		1440
• LuxIR Fractional handpiece		850–1350
Affirm	Cynosure	1320, 1440

With fractional non-ablative technologies, treatment columns are delivered about 300–1200 microns deep, in contrast to the typical 200–300-micron depth of multiple-pass CO_2 laser resurfacing [43]. A zone of normal skin surrounds each microscopic treatment column, leaving the barrier function of the epidermis intact without any visible wounding. The stratum corneum remains intact during and after laser firing. Patients can often apply makeup or sunscreen following treatment. The normal intervening tissue allows for rapid re-epithelialization by keratinocyte migration and division of transient amplifying cells into the treatment column. After 2–3 days, the tops of the wounded areas are shed as microscopic epidermal and dermal necrotic debris (MENDs) [44]. When there is disruption of the basement membrane, dermal as well as epidermal contents are expelled in the MENDs. Further collagen remodeling continues in the microthermal zone over the next 3–6 months. On average, each session treats about 20% of the skin surface, so between four and seven treatments are needed for optimal results. This is in contrast to the one to three treatments that are required with more aggressive fractional ablative resurfacing.

Studies on fractional photothermolysis for the treatment of periorbital rhytides revealed mild improvement in 12% of patients, noticeable improvement in 30%, and moderate to significant improvement in 54%, 1 month after four treatments. Rokhsar and Fitzpatrick treated ten cases of resistant melasma with fractional photothermolysis. After 4–6 treatment sessions, 60% of patients achieved 75–100% clearing and 30% had less than 25% improvement [45]. Anecdotal evidence has demonstrated fractional photothermolysis to be useful in the treatment of solar lentigines, overall skin texture, and dilated pores following a series of 3–5 treatment sessions. The device appears to work better on fine to moderate rhytides than it does on deeper lines. Perioral vertical rhytides are particularly resistant.

As with other lower-recovery-time procedures, rhytides are not improved to the same degree as they are with fractional ablative resurfacing.

Fractional photothermolysis has also been studied in the treatment of acne scars. Rahman *et al.* evaluated 53 atrophic scars, including acne scars, surgical scars, traumatic scars, and striae, treated at low and high energies. Ninety-two percent of subjects demonstrated at least some clinical improvement and 66% of subjects showed 50–100% improvement of their scars [46]. Geronemus and colleagues treated 17 subjects with ice-pick, boxcar, and rolling type acne scars with five treatments at 1- to 3-week intervals. Mean improvement in acne scarring measured by topographic imaging was found to be 22–62% [47,48].

Weiss and colleagues studied the Cynosure 1440 nm Affirm device, which utilizes a microarray of lenses delivering a 10-mm beam as hundreds of high-fluence beamlets interspersed with relatively uniform low-fluence background irradiation, for the treatment of superficial rhytides, scars, and photoaging [49]. Eighty-two percent of subjects exhibited mild to moderate improvement, and 12% exhibited good improvement. Side effects were minimal and included mild post-treatment erythema and edema resolving within 24 hours. Pain during treatment was judged minimal to moderate. Post-auricular histology showed areas of thermal injury up to 250 microns deep and 150 microns wide.

Conclusion

Compared to fractional ablative resurfacing techniques, non-ablative photo-rejuvenation, including fractional non-ablative treatments, offer milder clinical improvement, despite significant histological changes noted in multiple studies. On the other hand, patients generally experience minimal to no downtime following such treatments. Fractional non-ablative treatments clearly lead to better results than are seen with traditional non-ablative technologies, but more treatment sessions are required than with fractional ablative laser treatments.

References

1 Kauvar AN, Waldorf HA, Geronemus RG. A histopathological comparison of "char-free" carbon dioxide lasers. *Dermatol Surg* 1996; **22**: 343–8.
2 Cotton J, Hood AF, Gonin R, Beesen WH, Hanke CW. Histologic evaluation of preauricular and postauricular human skin after high-energy, short-pulse carbon dioxide laser. *Arch Dermatol* 1996; **132**: 425–8.
3 Krane SM. The importance of proline residues in the structure, stability and susceptibility to proteolytic degradation of collagens. *Amino Acids* 2008; **35**: 703–10.

4 Verzar F, Nagy IZ. Electronmicroscopic analysis of thermal collagen denaturation in rat tail tendons. *Gerontologia* 1970; **16**: 77–82.

5 Nagy IZ, Toth VN, Verzar F. High-resolution electron microscopy of thermal collagen denaturation in tail tendons of young, adult and old rats. *Connect Tissue Res* 1974; **2**: 265–72.

6 Goldberg DJ. Non-ablative subsurface remodeling: clinical and histologic evaluation of a 1320-nm Nd:YAG laser. *J Cutan Laser Ther* 1999; **1**: 153–7.

7 Mordon S, Capon A, Creusy C, *et al.* In vivo experimental evaluation of skin remodeling by using an Er:Glass laser with contact cooling. *Lasers Surg Med* 2000; **27**: 1–9.

8 Wade TR, Wade SL, Jones HE. Skin changes and diseases associated with pregnancy. *Obstet Gynecol* 1978; **52**: 233–42.

9 Roenigk HH, Pinski JB, Robinson JK, Hanke CW. Acne, retinoids, and dermabrasion. *J Dermatol Surg Oncol* 1985; **11**: 396–8.

10 Rubenstein R, Roenigk HH, Stegman SJ, Hanke CW. Atypical keloids after dermabrasion of patients taking isotretinoin. *J Am Acad Dermatol* 1986; **15**: 280–5.

11 Zachariae H. Delayed wound healing and keloid formation following argon laser treatment or dermabrasion during isotretinoin treatment. *Br J Dermatol* 1988; **118**: 703–6.

12 Semchyshyn NL, Kilmer SL. Does laser inactivate botulinum toxin? *Dermatol Surg* 2005; **31**: 399–404.

13 Goldman MP, Alster TS, Weiss R. A randomized trial to determine the influence of laser therapy, monopolar radiofrequency treatment, and intense pulsed light therapy administered immediately after hyaluronic acid gel implantation. *Dermatol Surg* 2007; **33**: 535–42.

14 Bitter PH. Noninvasive rejuvenation of photodamaged skin using serial, full-face intense pulsed light treatments. *Dermatol Surg* 2000; **26**: 835–42.

15 Weiss RA, Weiss MA, Beasley KL. Rejuvenation of photoaged skin: 5 years results with intense pulsed light of the face, neck, and chest. *Dermatol Surg* 2002; **28**: 1115–19.

16 Sadick NS, Weiss R, Kilmer S, Bitter P. Photorejuvenation with intense pulsed light: results of a multi-center study. *J Drugs Dermatol* 2004; **3**: 41–9.

17 Goldberg DJ. New collagen formation after dermal remodeling with an intense pulsed light source. *J Cutan Laser Ther* 2000; **2**: 59–61.

18 Negishi K, Wakamatsu S, Kushikata N, Tezuka Y, Kotani Y, Shiba K. Full-face photorejuvenation of photodamaged skin by intense pulsed light with integrated contact cooling: initial experiences in Asian patients. *Lasers Surg Med* 2002; **30**: 298–305.

19 Hernandez-Perez E, Ibiett EV. Gross and microscopic findings in patients submitted to nonablative full face resurfacing using intense pulsed light. *Dermatol Surg* 2002; **28**: 651–5.

20 Anderson RR, Parish JA. Selective photothermolysis: precise microsurgery by selective absorption of pulsed radiation. *Science* 1983; **220**: 524–7.

21 Goldberg DJ, Samady JA. Intense pulsed light and Nd:YAG laser nonablative treatment of facial rhytids. *Lasers Surg Med* 2001; **28**: 141–4.

22 Negishi K, Tezuka Y, Kushikata N, Wakamatsu S. Photorejuvenation for Asian skin by intense pulsed light. *Dermatol Surg* 2001; **27**: 627–31.

23 Ross EV. Laser versus intense pulsed light: competing technologies in dermatology. *Lasers Surg Med* 2006; **38**: 261–72.

24 Khoury JG, Goldman MP. Use of light-emitting diode photomodulation to reduce erythema and discomfort after intense pulsed light treatment of photodamage. *J Cosmet Dermatol* 2008; **7**: 30–4.

25 Goldman MP, Weiss RA, Weiss MA. Intense pulsed light as a nonablative approach to photoaging. *Dermatol Surg* 2005; **31**: 1179–87.

26 Goldberg DJ, Cutler KB. Nonablative treatment of rhytids with intense pulsed light. *Lasers Surg Med* 2000; **26**: 196–200.

27 Negishi K, Kushikata N, Takeuchi K, Tezuka Y, Wakamatsu S. Photorejuvenation by intense pulsed light with objective measurement of skin color in Japanese patients. *Dermatol Surg* 2006; **32**: 1380–7.

28 Hardaway CA, Ross EV, Barnette DJ, Paithankar DY. (2002) Non-ablative cutaneous remodeling with a 1.45 microm mid-infrared diode laser: phase I. *J Cosmet Laser Ther* 2002; **4**: 3–8.

29 Dang Y, Ren Q, Liu H, Ma J, Zhang J. Effects of the 1320-nm Nd:YAG laser on transepidermal water loss, histological changes, and collagen remodeling in skin. *Lasers Med Sci* 2006; **21**: 147–52.

30 Lupton JR, Williams CM, Alster TS. Nonablative laser skin resurfacing using a 1540 nm erbium glass laser: a clinical and histologic analysis. *Dermatol Surg* 2002; **28**: 833–5.

31 Trelles MA. Short and long-term follow-up of nonablative 1320 nm Nd:YAG laser facial rejuvenation. *Dermatol Surg* 2001; **27**: 781–2.

32 Fatemi A, Weiss MA, Weiss RA. Short-term histologic effects of nonablative resurfacing: results with a dynamically cooled millisecond-domain 1320 nm Nd:YAG laser. *Dermatol Surg* 2002; **28**: 172–6.

33 Orringer JS, Voorhees JJ, Hamilton T, *et al*. Dermal matrix remodeling after nonablative laser therapy. *J Am Acad Dermatol* 2005; **53**: 775–82.

34 Kelly KM, Nelson JS, Lask GP, Geronemus RG, Bernstein LJ. Cryogen spray cooling in combination with nonablative laser treatment of facial rhytides. *Arch Dermatol* 1999; **135**: 691–4.

35 Lupton JR, Alster TS. Nonablative cutaneous laser resurfacing using a 1.54 microm erbium-doped phosphate glass laser: a clinical and histologic study. *Lasers Surg Med* 2001; (Suppl 13): S46.

36 Fournier N, Dahan S, Barneon G, *et al*. Nonablative remodeling: clinical, histologic, ultrasound imaging, and profilometric evaluation of a 1540 nm Er:glass laser. *Dermatol Surg* 2001; **27**: 799–806.

37 Fournier N, Dahan S, Barneon G, *et al*. Nonablative remodeling: a 14-month clinical ultrasound imaging and profilometric evaluation of a 1540 nm Er:Glass laser. *Dermatol Surg* 2001; **28**: 926–31.

38 Goldberg DJ, Rogachefsky AS, Silapunt S. Non-ablative laser treatment of facial rhytides: a comparison of 1450-nm diode laser treatment with dynamic cooling as opposed to treatment with dynamic cooling alone. *Lasers Surg Med* 2002; **30**: 79–81.

39 Tanzi EL, Williams CM, Alster TS. Treatment of facial rhytides with a nonablative 1450-nm diode laser: a controlled clinical and histologic study. *Dermatol Surg* 2003; **29**: 124–8.

40 Chan HH, Lam LK, Wong DS, Kono T, Trendell-Smith N. Use of 1320 nm Nd:YAG laser for wrinkle reduction and the treatment of atrophic acne scarring in Asians. *Lasers Surg Med* 2004; **34**: 98–103.

41 Hardaway CA, Ross EV, Paithankar DY. Non-ablative cutaneous remodeling with a 1.45 microm mid-infrared diode laser: phase II. *J Cosmet Laser Ther* 2002; **4**: 9–14.

42 Manstein D, Herron GS, Sink RK, Tanner H, Anderson RR. Fractional photothermolysis: a new concept for cutaneous remodeling using microscopic patterns of thermal injury. *Lasers Surg Med* 2004; **34**: 426–38.

43 Laubach H, Tannous Z, Anderson RR, Manstein D. A histological evaluation of the dermal effects after fractional photothermolysis treatment. *Lasers Surg Med* 2005; **36** (Suppl 17): 86.

44 Tannous Z, Laubach HJ, Anderson RR, Manstein D. Changes of epidermal pigment distribution after fractional resurfacing: a clinicopathologic correlation. *Lasers Surg Med* 2005; **36** (Suppl 17): 32.

45 Rokhsar CK, Fitzpatrick RE. The treatment of melasma with fractional photothermolysis: a pilot study. *Dermatol Surg* 2005; **31**: 1645–50.

46 Rahman Z, Tanner H, Jiang K. Treatment of atrophic scars with the 1550 nm erbium-fiber fractional laser. *Lasers Surg Med* 2006; **38** (Suppl 18): 24.

47 Geronemus RG. Fractional photothermolysis: current and future applications. *Lasers Surg Med* 2006; **38**: 169–76.

48 Kim KH, Fisher GH, Bernstein L, Bangesh S, Skover G, Geronemus R. Treatment of acneiform scars with fractional photothermolysis. *Lasers Surg Med* 2005; **36** (Suppl 17): 31.

49 Weiss RA, Bene NI, Weiss MA, Beasley KL. Long term clinical trial of 1440 nm combined apex pulse array laser for treatment of scars and rhytides. *Lasers Surg Med* 2007; **39** (Suppl 19): 82.

CHAPTER 3

Fractional Ablative Resurfacing

Joshua A. Tournas and Christopher B. Zachary
University of California at Irvine, CA, USA

Key points
- Initial ablative laser resurfacing devices were non-fractionated
- Today's fractional ablative devices have replaced the older systems
- Fractional ablative devices are categorized as carbon dioxide, erbium, and erbium:YSGG
- Complications may be seen even with today's safer fractional ablative lasers

---

Introduction

The use of ablative (carbon dioxide and erbium) lasers for facial resurfacing fell out of favor in the early 2000s as less aggressive devices promising results with no major aftercare proliferated. Although they delivered on the promise of no "downtime," they suffered from a lack of efficacy. As the concept of fractional photothermolysis matured, it has been adapted to the aforementioned ablative laser wavelengths, leading to a new class of lasers, termed "fractional ablative." Numerous devices have since debuted, which offer efficacy that is well above that of the non-ablative lasers, and with a much lower overall risk profile than the original ablative devices. Initially fractional non-ablative devices replaced the standard non-ablative devices as technologies that led to improvement but required many treatment sessions. These are now being replaced, in many instances, with fractional ablative devices.

Background

The use of lasers in cosmetic surgery traces its roots back to the first uses of the continuous-wave carbon dioxide (CO_2) laser for skin resurfacing in the early 1990s [1–8], and their use has since expanded into the large and diverse market we have today. With these early devices, considerable correction of the signs of photoaging such as rhytides, laxity, and dyschromia were easily

---

Facial Resurfacing, 1st edition. Edited by David J. Goldberg. © 2010 Blackwell Publishing.

seen, although the healing time was quite protracted. Given that the entire epidermis and superficial dermis are ablated and coagulated to a depth of approximately 150–300 microns with such procedures, meticulous post-operative care with numerous dressing changes was necessary. Recovery time can be troublesome, is generally uncomfortable, and can take from 2 weeks to a month; and patients can be left with significant erythema, which can persist for 3–6 months. Even in the hands of the expert laser surgeon, unfortunate patients might develop scarring, noticeable lines of demarcation, and delayed-onset permanent hypopigmentation [9]. While the use of traditional fully ablative CO_2 and erbuim:YAG lasers for skin resurfacing is still seen, the above-mentioned issues have relegated these devices to a much smaller group of laser surgeons with the expertise to perform such treatments and the willingness to risk potential adverse effects with their use.

With the turn of the twenty-first century, frustration on the part of physicians and patients with the hazards of fully ablative resurfacing led to the development of a new class of aesthetic devices which were termed "non-ablative." A variety of technologies utilizing 1064, 1320, and 1540 nm lasers, radiofrequency, intense pulsed light (IPL), and combined devices were adapted to this purpose [10]. Whatever the method of delivery, the goal was to provide bulk dermal heating that would cause collagen denaturation and then remodeling, all the while protecting the epidermis with a cooling mechanism. These procedures were associated with lower risk, limited healing time with modest edema, and erythema lasting 1–2 days, but reduced efficacy. Research and development is ongoing, but continued experience with this class of device has led many to conclude that they are of limited usefulness for the treatment of skin laxity and rhytides. Meanwhile, there remains no doubt that IPLs can provide tremendous improvement in dyschromia and vascularity.

The concept of "fractional photothermolysis" saw its debut with the Fraxel device (now called Fraxel re:store; Solta Medical, Hayward, CA). This device is uses a 1550 nm erbium-glass laser and a scanning handpiece to lay down rows of narrow laser pulses (on the order of 150–200 microns wide), creating "microthermal zones" of heated tissue surrounded by intact skin. Multiple other lasers operating in this wavelength range (1440–1550 nm) have been introduced, the main difference between them being the method of delivery, rather than the concept behind it. The selective heating of these extremely narrow columns of tissue allows spectacularly high fluences to create cylindrical areas of damaged tissue, each surrounded by intact epidermis and dermis to provide structure and nutritional support during the recovery phase. These devices, which will be referred to henceforth as "fractional non-ablative lasers" have taken a pre-eminent stance in the facial rejuvenation armamentarium, with indications such as rhytides, dyschromia, acne scarring, and melasma [11].

Given the strong performance of the fractional non-ablative laser class over the past 5 years, it should not be surprising to note that researchers and the laser industry would surmise that the technique of "fractionation" could be implemented with wavelengths other than the existing infrared devices. Specifically, work began in 2005 with the 10 600 nm carbon dioxide (CO_2) laser and soon extended to the 2940 nm erbium:YAG (Er:YAG) laser. Referred to in early studies as "fractional deep dermal ablation" [12–16], these devices used concepts similar to those described above, but with the ablative wavelengths. It was thought that by using fractional techniques the skin could be treated to much greater depths than previously possible without the complications associated with fully ablative lasers, and with much shorter recovery times.

Early studies that helped form the concept of fractional ablative resurfacing were performed by manually modulating a standard CO_2 laser to create narrow columns of destruction for subsequent hair transplantation, as well as in the treatment of syringomas, both using laser pulses of approximately 1 mm beam diameter. While fractional ablative resurfacing is not used for hair transplantation or for the treatment of syringomata, the fact that in both cases the wounds healed without scarring launched inquiry into just how effective this type of device could be for cosmetic indications. Further in vitro and in vivo study delineated the concept further. While traditional ablative lasers remove the entire epidermis and dermis to a shallow depth, the fractional ablative lasers vaporize narrow columns of tissue to a significant depth (1–1.5 mm), inducing not only "resurfacing" but also "volumetric tissue reduction," whereby each treatment ejects a certain volume of cutaneous tissue, with significant horizontal contraction reducing the final overall surface area of treated skin [12,13].

The next section will detail the various fractional ablative laser devices available at the time of writing. While the authors prefer the term "fractional" be applied to devices which create pulses that are deeper than they are wide, some variation on this concept exists. Therefore, in the interest of completeness, devices will be included which might rather fit a broader definition of the term.

Fractional ablative devices

CO_2 devices

Fraxel re:pair
The Fraxel re:pair laser system (Solta Medical, Hayward, CA) was the first entrant into the fractional ablative arena, combining some features of the

original Fraxel laser (now marketed as Fraxel re:store) with the 10 600 nm CO_2 laser wavelength. The handpiece uses a scanning mechanism that senses movement across the skin surface and will only deliver its strip-like pattern of laser pulses when the treatment head is in motion. The energy delivered with each pulse and the overall density of pulses can be adjusted by the user, and the device reports the approximate treatment depth to be expected with the given settings. The histology of the delivered laser pulses has been well characterized, ranging from 120 to 150 microns wide, and over 1500 microns in depth [12,13].

New handpieces have recently been developed, including a "pseudo-fractional" handpiece, providing laser pulses that are 600 microns wide and approximately 100–200 microns in depth, a 0.2 mm incisional handpiece, and a 2 mm standard ablative handpiece.

Lumenis DeepFX/ActiveFX

The Lumenis DeepFX and ActiveFX handpieces (Lumenis Inc., Santa Clara, CA) are extensions of the company's existing UltraPulse Encore CO_2 laser platform, which also includes ablative and incisional handpieces. The ActiveFX handpiece uses a computer pattern generator (CPG) to deliver an array of pseudo-fractional laser pulses that are 1.25 mm wide and approximately 200–300 microns in depth, in patterns that are distracted, one from the other. Pulses are laid down in a random rather than sequential pattern to avoid bulk heating.

In contrast to the ActiveFX handpiece, the DeepFX handpiece released in late 2007 is a true fractional device, providing laser pulses that are approximately 120 microns wide and over 1500 microns in depth. This is a stamp-type device, which has recently been upgraded to provide faster generation of pulses in a raster-scan pattern rather than the former concentrically arranged pattern of pulses. Handpieces can also now be exchanged without powering down the laser system. The parameters are such that this device should be very comparable clinically with the Fraxel re:pair, though with slower scanning speeds.

Lutronic eCO_2

The Lutronic eCO_2 laser (Lutronic USA, Princeton Junction, NJ) is built on a 30 watt CO_2 laser platform, and offers a variety of treatment options. Spot sizes of 120, 180, and 300 microns are available to the user, and the manufacturer reports that penetration depths up to 2.5 mm using the 120 micron spot size are possible. The maximum area covered by the scanner is 14 mm × 14 mm, and spots can be delivered in rectangular, circular, and triangular shapes. User-controlled factors include the spot size, scan area size, pulse energy, and density of spots (25–400 spots/cm^2). The treatment pattern can also be delivered in an ordered, raster-scan fashion or in a random pattern, termed "controlled chaos technology."

SmartXide DOT

The SmartXide DOT laser device (Eclipsemed, Inc., Dallas, TX) is also based on a 30 watt continuous-wave CO_2 laser. The DOT delivers laser energy into the tissue in spots 350 microns wide, placing it in squarely between true fractional devices such as the Fraxel re:pair (135 microns) and larger-spot "pseudo-fractional" devices such as the ActiveFX (1250 microns, or 1.25 mm). The treatment pattern is 15 mm × 15 mm. User-controlled parameters for this device are the laser's dwell time (0.2–2.0 ms) and the distance between adjacent spots (0.2–1.0 mm). The maximal energy per pulse is 60 mJ, which over a 350 micron spot provides depths that should be relatively shallow and quick to heal, but this has not been fully characterized in the literature. As with many of the other devices in this category, the DOT laser offers standard non-fractional handpieces as well.

Lasering Mixto SX/Candela QuadraLase

The Mixto SX (Lasering USA Inc., San Ramon, CA), also marketed as the QuadraLase (Candela, Inc., Wayland, WA), is another fractional device built on a standard CO_2 laser platform that produces a scanned pattern of spots that are 300 microns wide in a scan area ranging from 6 mm × 6 mm to 20 mm × 20 mm. According to the manufacturer, the depth of the spots varies from 20 to 500 microns, and treatment density can be varied from 20% to 100%. User-controlled parameters are the output wattage of the continuous-wave laser and the "SX index", which represents the "dwell time" of the continuous-wave laser at each treatment spot, with the logical conclusion being that a longer dwell time results in a greater depth of injury.

Alma Pixel CO_2

The Pixel CO_2 device (Alma Lasers, Inc., Buffalo Grove, IL) is a stand-alone fractional ablative device based on a 30 watt continuous-wave CO_2 laser. Similar to the manufacturer's Pixel Er:YAG device described below, two patterns of spots are available – square patterns containing either 49 (7 × 7) or 81 (9 × 9) spots or "pixels." Unlike many of the other devices, the Pixel devices use a beam splitter to deliver the entirety of the fractional pattern with a single laser pulse rather than using a scanning mechanism. Surgical handpieces are also offered. A separate handpiece, the Pixel CO_2 Omnifit, is also available, employing similar beam-splitting technology, and this can be adapted to other existing CO_2 laser platforms from other manufacturers to produce a similar effect to the Pixel CO_2 device.

Erbium:YAG devices

Sciton ProFractional
The Sciton ProFractional device (Sciton, Inc., Palo Alto, CA) is a 2940 nm erbium:YAG fractional handpiece which operates on either their Profile or their newer Joule platform. This device has a scanning-type handpiece with a 2 cm × 2 cm window, and the user can treat 1.5–60% of the skin with 400-micron spots. Large and small treatment areas are selectable as well, and the maximum depth of the fractional spots is 1200 microns. With the ProFractional, the user selects the desired depth of penetration and density, and the device calculates the necessary fluence. The ProFractional-XC handpiece is a further modification which allows the user to add a variable amount of coagulation to the ablative pulse, bringing the effect of this device closer to what is seen with the CO_2-based devices, as well as faster scanning speed.

Palomar Lux2940
The Palomar Lux2940 device (Palomar Medical Technologies, Burlington, MA) incorporates an Er:YAG handpiece which mounts on the manufacturer's StarLux platform. Similar to the Sciton and Alma, this allows a single unit to house multiple devices including intense pulsed light, fractional non-ablative, and fractional ablative. The Lux2940 can deliver up to 1000 "microbeams"/cm^2 over either a 10 mm × 10 mm or 6 mm × 6 mm area. This device also delivers pulses in pure-ablative, coagulative, or blended modes, and the theoretical maximum treatment depth is over 1 mm. Early studies on this device showed rapid re-epithelization in 12 hours, and treatment depths of approximately 250 microns with typical settings [17].

Alma Pixel Er:YAG
The Alma Pixel 2940 device (Alma Lasers, Buffalo Grove, IL) is a 2940 nm Er:YAG handpiece that operates on the company's Harmony platform. The Pixel delivers 49 or 81 (7 × 7 or 9 × 9) laser spots or "pixels," using a beam splitter within a single 11 mm × 11 mm square treatment field, much as with the Pixel CO_2 device discussed above. The pulse energy is therefore divided among either the 49 or 81 spots, such that the 49-pixel pattern will result in fewer but deeper spots while the 81-pixel pattern will create more spots, but they will not be as deep. The width of each spot is approximately 50 microns, and the depth of penetration is 20–50 microns, resulting in a superficial peeling effect. A multiple-pass technique with this device has also been characterized, which causes vacuolar damage and superficial elimination of epidermis, as well as mild residual thermal effect [18]. Another study with the Pixel device showed histological evidence of diffuse new collagen formation as far out as 2 months after treatment [19]. A higher-power

version of this device was recently developed, the High Power Pixel 2940. This updated handpiece offers similar treatments as the original Pixel, but at depths up to 150 microns.

YSGG devices

Cutera Pearl Fractional

The Cutera Pearl Fractional device (Cutera, Inc., Brisbane, CA) utilizes an erbium:yttrium-scandium-gallium-garnet (Er:YSGG) laser with a wavelength of 2790 nm that primarily targets water, much like Er:YAG and CO_2 devices. The YSGG wavelength has slightly less water absorption than the 2940 Er:YAG device, and slightly more coagulative effect. This device delivers 300-micron diameter columns that penetrate 300–1500 microns with 40–60 microns of surrounding thermal damage. Early results have indicated treatment results similar to those seen with Er:YAG devices. The platform also supports a standard fully ablative Er:YSGG handpiece. A recent study by Ross *et al.* described ablation at depth up to 80 microns with the fully ablative Pearl device [20].

Treatment techniques

Patient selection

As will be discussed below, the treatment indications for fractional ablative laser treatment are broad, but common concepts abound in patient selection. One should seek to treat patients with manageable conditions combined with reasonable expectations as well as compatible skin types.

The initial expectation that a single fractional ablative treatment might provide results approximating those of traditional CO_2 laser with a fraction of the downtime have not necessarily been realized. To be sure, these devices provide excellent results, and the downtime is certainly shortened. However, results have been somewhat less predictable than with fully ablative devices, and while good results are achievable with a single treatment, in our experience many conditions require multiple-treatment protocols. With respect to rhytides, patients with fine-to-moderate wrinkling and periorbital rhytides tend to respond considerably better than those with deeper lines and excessive laxity around the perioral area. This is not to say that those with deeper lines should not be treated, but rather that the amount of improvement to be expected (especially with a single treatment) is certainly less. There has been a general trend in our patients toward desiring an age-appropriate "freshened" and "rejuvenated" appearance. Many of the patients seen in warmer areas will have worse-than-expected photodamage for their age. It is in this middle-aged but considerably weathered population that the results of these procedures can most readily be seen. Patients expecting near-total elimination of rhytides should be steered toward fully ablative laser procedures or surgical management.

The use of fully ablative devices has been restricted by some to those patients with lighter skin phototypes (generally Fitzpatrick types I–II), or they have been used very cautiously and much less aggressively in patients with darker skin [21], to avoid post-inflammatory hyperpigmentation. However, it has been our experience that patients with darker phototypes can be safely treated with fully ablative laser devices, given appropriate precautions which will be discussed below. In practice, we routinely treat patients with darker skin types, most commonly for acne scars.

Pre-treatment preparation

Patients undergoing laser treatment of any type in our clinic are made aware at the time of consultation of the potential risks of laser treatment, such as scarring, hyper- or hypopigmentation, and milia/acne formation. Specifically with regard to ablative or fractional ablative laser treatment, this discussion is expanded to include the concept of "downtime," and the need for meticulous skin care in the immediate post-treatment period. While fractional ablative treatment certainly provides for a much-reduced downtime, serosanguinous discharge is common and crusting is avoided by regular vinegar soaks and the application of moisturizers on a regular basis. Most patients will be able to apply makeup or otherwise attend social functions in 4–7 days, depending on depth and density of treatment. Patients are given ample opportunity to ask questions of the physician during the consultation and again when reviewing the preoperative and postoperative instructions with the nursing staff afterward. Patients are counseled to have a companion available to drive them home post-procedure.

Patients are questioned as to their medical and surgical history, including other cosmetic procedures and medications. Patients who have a history of connective tissue disease, those who have taken oral retinoids within the last year, and those with a history of keloid scars are excluded from treatment due to the risk of scarring. Caution should also be exercised in those who have had prior resurfacing procedures or blepharoplasty, and in those who smoke [1]. Patients are not routinely provided a regimen to condition the skin before treatment, other than aggressive sun avoidance and sunscreen use.

As is the case with fully ablative laser treatments, infection is a significant concern with the fractional ablative lasers due to epidermal disruption. While large case series are lacking in this laser class, there have been anecdotal reports of viral (mainly herpes simplex), bacterial, and fungal infections of the skin in the postoperative period. With traditional CO_2 resurfacing, infection rates approaching 10% have been documented without prophylaxis

[22,23]. In our practice, we provide every patient with prescriptions for oral prophylactic medication to start the day of the procedure for viral, bacterial, and fungal infection regardless of prior infection history or herpes simplex virus (HSV) status as follows:

- acyclovir 400 mg three times daily × 14 days
- cephalexin 500 mg twice daily × 7 days
- fluconazole 200 mg daily × 4 days

Having said this, many physicians will just offer the antivirals as prophylaxis.

Post-inflammatory hyperpigmentation is a significant concern in darker skin types, and will occur in nearly 100% of these patients without intervention. For patients with type III or darker skin, we prescribe 4% hydroquinone to be applied topically twice daily starting immediately after the cessation of serosanguinous discharge in the postoperative period. Those patients with a prior history of melasma or other pigmentary disorders are generally started on hydroquinone at least 1 month prior to treatment.

Day-of-procedure considerations

Patients undergoing fractional ablative resurfacing in our practice are asked to arrive approximately 1 hour prior to the planned treatment time for preoperative preparation and anesthesia. The face and the neck (if being treated) are thoroughly washed with a mild cleanser.

Following thorough cleansing, a topical anesthetic agent is applied. In our practice, patients have consistently received a mixture of 23% lidocaine and 7% tetracaine in a lipophilic ointment for 1 hour. Adjunctive anesthesia, however, has undergone considerable evolution. In the authors' earliest clinical trial experience with the fractional CO_2 laser, oral hydrocodone/acetaminophen and lorazepam were used, although pain control was not found to be suboptimal [14]. Later studies used a combination of topical anesthesia with nerve blocks. 1% lidocaine with 1:100 000 epinephrine was used to perform regional blocks of the supraorbital, supratrochlear, infraorbital, mental, zygomaticotemporal and zygomaticofacial nerve trunks bilaterally [16]. This was augmented with local infiltration in some areas if particularly aggressive treatment was planned. However, our current practice for full-face and/or neck treatments is a combination of intramuscular injections of meperidine (Demerol), hydroxyzine (Vistaril), and toradol given approximately 30 minutes prior to the start of the laser procedure. This has proven more effective than nerve blocks and better-tolerated by the patient. Some patients receive 6 mg intramuscular betamethasone suspension (Celestone Soluspan) to reduce postoperative swelling. However, recent practice is to apply potent topical steriod cream immediately after the procedure, as this significantly reduces the bleeding and seepage.

Unlike most traditional CO_2 and Er:YAG devices, most of the available fractional ablative laser devices have handpieces that come in contact with the skin as the laser energy is being delivered. That said, it is still prudent to prepare the treatment field with damp surgical towels to prevent ignition of flammable substances surrounding the patient. Surgical personnel involved in the procedure should don "laser-grade" surgical masks, and it is imperative that a suction unit be used, whether it is built into the unit or stand-alone. For patients whose eyelids will be treated, steel corneal shields are employed.

Intraoperatively, a forced cold air device (Zimmer Cryo 6, Zimmer, Inc., Irvine, CA) is used to augment the aforementioned anesthetic measures. Once topical anesthetic is removed from the area to be treated, a "striping" or "stamping" pattern is employed to lay down the requisite density of ablated columns of tissue. Although we previously used a 50% overlap technique, we now avoid any immediate overlap because of the potential for bulk heating with the former technique. Subsequent stripes, both parallel and at right angles, are laid down so as to create an even application of microablative zones. With devices using a stamping pattern, overlap is generally not employed, and the density of spots desired can generally be delivered in one pass.

Treatment pearls

Regardless of the device or treatment pattern, there are some common techniques to use, and pitfalls to avoid. While lines of demarcation are not seen as commonly with the fractional ablative lasers as with previous fully ablative devices, one should take care to avoid gaps in treatment. For stripe-type devices, this is commonly avoided by applying at least four passes, divided horizontally and vertically. Stamp-type devices can show this effect when the "stamps" are placed too far apart from one another. Careful inspection as the treatment concludes can often illuminate these areas, and they can be treated in a low-energy, low-density fashion to complete the pattern with minimal risk of overtreatment.

Once the treatment is complete, feathering can be employed to further camouflage the transition from facial to neck skin, and from treated to untreated skin. Typically the pulse energy is reduced to near-minimum levels, and passes completed around the lateral cheeks, mandible, and, if the neck is treated, the upper chest and lateral neck. This technique is also useful when only treating a portion of the face, such as in a young patient with acne scarring limited to the cheeks.

The ability to treat the neck is a large advantage of the fractional ablative lasers over earlier devices, though this requires much lower pulse energies and density of pulses. We generally limit the energy to about 30 mJ per pulse using the Fraxel re:pair device, and with no more that 20% density.

Post-treatment care

Immediately after treatment, patients will often have serosanguinous discharge and/or pinpoint bleeding, especially when using devices that offer less coagulation. Gentle cleansing with saline solution and soft gauze is employed to cleanse the face, removing any dried tissue fluid or blood that is present after treatment. Once clean, a potent topical steroid cream is applied. For deeper treatments that are more likely to produce post-treatment discharge, topical zinc oxide paste can be applied. If lower-energy treatments are employed, the risk of post-treatment acneiform eruptions is greatly reduced, and petrolatum-based occlusive emollients may be used immediately post-treatment. Patients are reminded to sleep flat with their head elevated, and to use old bed linens that can be disposed of if soiled.

The hallmark of good post-treatment care after fractional ablative resurfacing is the avoidance of crusting. In earliest studies, patients who meticulously cared for their skin post-treatment healed faster and were re-engaged in work or social activities sooner than those who did so to a lesser extent [14]. To that end, patients are instructed to remove their emollient with gentle cleanser and a soft washcloth three to five times daily, or as dictated by their level of serosanguinous discharge, and then to use compresses with a dilute solution of 10:1 bottled or distilled water to 5% acetic acid solution (vinegar soaks), applied to the treated areas for 10–15 minutes, followed by gentle wiping of any loosened crust without any scrubbing, and reapplication of the emollient. Once the discharge and any crust have subsided, changing to a petrolatum-based emollient or similar product will speed the return to work or other social activity. Patients should return for frequent re-checks to assess their healing and self-care, with adjustments as necessary.

Indications and outcomes

Rhytides and photoaging

Multiple studies have detailed the effectiveness of fractional ablative resurfacing in improving the changes of photoaging (Figs. 3.1–3.5). Rahman *et al.* [14] reported a two-part study, the first phase of which treated 24 patients with a prototype of what is now the Fraxel re:pair device at settings of 5–40 mJ per pulse, 400 microthermal zones (MTZ) per cm^2 on the forearm with clinical and histologic evaluation at 1 and 3 months post-treatment. These early studies indicated that erythema and edema did not persist as judged by the 3-month follow-up visit. Following this initial study, 30 patients were treated once or twice with the same prototype device, 5–40 mJ per pulse, 400–1200 MTZ/cm^2. Independent investigators rated improvements as greater than 50% in rhytides, pigmentation, texture, and vascular lesions, and 26–50% improved in laxity. Average improvement in Fitzpatrick wrinkle score (0–9 scale) was 1.47. Post-inflammatory hyper-pigmentation was observed transiently in six patients. Erythema was seen

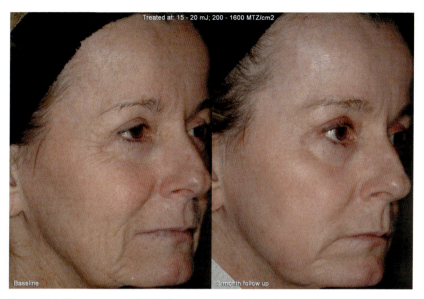

Figure 3.1 Photodamage: (left) before treatment; (right) showing improvement 3 months after fractional ablative laser resurfacing.

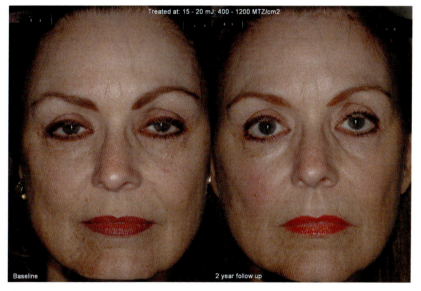

Figure 3.2 Photodamage: (left) before treatment; (right) showing improvement 2 years after fractional ablative laser resurfacing.

postoperatively in all patients, persisting in ten patients at 1 month, and at 3 months in two patients. Delayed-onset hypopigmentation was not observed. Clementoni *et al.* published a series of 55 patients treated with ActiveFX, evaluated at 1 and 3 months [24]. Patients received a single-pass

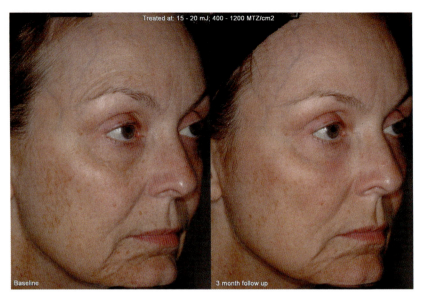

Figure 3.3 Photodamage: (left) before treatment; (right) showing improvement 3 months after fractional ablative laser resurfacing.

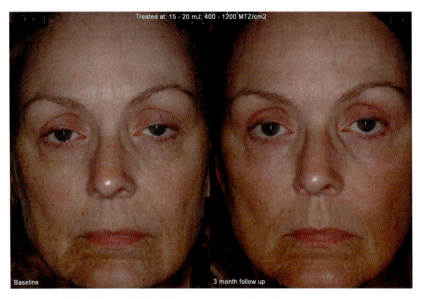

Figure 3.4 Photodamage: (left) before treatment; (right) showing improvement 3 months after fractional ablative laser resurfacing.

treatment with 100 mJ pulses, resulting in approximately 80-micron ablation with 200 microns of further thermal damage. Significant improvement was seen on quartile scale in global, fine lines, mottled pigment, sallowness, texture, but not coarse wrinkles or telangectasias. Mean healing time was

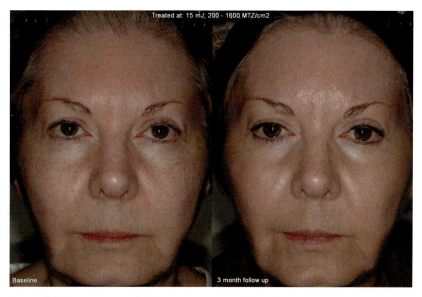

Figure 3.5 Photodamage: (left) before treatment; (right) showing improvement 3 months after fractional ablative laser resurfacing.

3.3 days, and erythema lasted a mean of 13.6 days. Berlin *et al.* also recently reported a series of ten patients ranging in age from 40 to 69 with type I–III skin who were treated with one single-pass full-face ActiveFX treatment [25]. Improvements in rhytides, elastosis, and texture on a five-point scale on blinded investigator analysis averaged 1.8 at 4 weeks, and 1.6 at 24 weeks, with patient satisfaction rating slightly higher. Histology showed decreased solar elastosis, and electron microscopy showed decreased collagen fibril diameter, consistent with increased type III collagen deposition. No delayed hypopigmentation was observed.

Acne scarring

Two prospective studies have been published using a fractional CO_2 laser for the treatment of acne scarring (Figs. 3.6–3.10). Chapas *et al.* [15] reported a study of 13 subjects with type I–IV skin and moderate-to-severe acne scarring who received two to three treatments with a prototype of the Fraxel re:pair device. Pulse energies ranged from 20 to 100 mJ, and densities from 200 to 1200 MTZ/cm². Density was reduced over sensitive areas. Erythema, edema, texture, atrophy, and overall improvement were graded on a quartile scale after each treatment and at 1 and 3 months' follow-up from the final treatment. Optical profilometry was performed on ten scars from each cheek on each patient. Clinical improvement of at least 26–50% on the quartile scales was noted in all patients, and the level of improvement on the optical scans ranged from 43% to 79.9%. Transient post-inflammatory

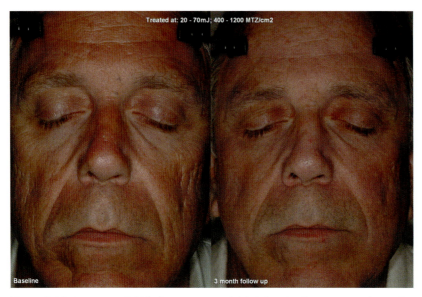

Figure 3.10 Acne scars: (left) before treatment; (right) showing improvement 3 months after fractional ablative laser resurfacing.

texture, 1.22 for atrophy, and 1.42 for overall appearance, with subject ratings averaging slightly higher.

Traumatic, surgical, and hypertrophic scars

Bolstered by the successful treatment of acne scarring with the fractional ablative lasers, multiple groups have attempted to treat other types of scarring as well. Cohen and Babcock recently reported a case of ice pick scarring in the nasal alar grooves from 1064 nm Nd:YAG treatment of facial telangectasias that was treated with the Sciton ProFractional fractional Er:YAG laser [26]. Three sessions at modest settings (175–350 micron depth, 3–4% coverage each treatment) were employed after unsuccessful treatment with a fractional non-ablative device. Waibel and Beer also recently published a case of a 50-year-old facial scar from a third-degree burn with subsequent improvement in texture and coloration using a combination of the Lumenis ActiveFX and DeepFX devices in a single treatment [27]. Gotkin *et al.* used the SmartXide DOT laser in a series of 32 patients aged 33–76 for various indications on the face, neck, trunk, and extremities, with pulse energies ranging from 10 to 60 mJ per pulse and spacing between spots from 200 to 800 microns [28]. Patients treated for scars and striae saw approximately 50% improvement as rated by an independent evaluator.

Melasma and post-inflammatory hyperpigmentation

While multiple studies have indicated there is a risk of post-inflammatory pigmentation or exacerbation of pre-existing pigmentary conditions with these devices at fluences used for treatment of rhytides and scars, work is ongoing in our center and others in an attempt to optimize treatment protocols for such problems. Very low-energy and low-density treatments have shown some promise and warrant further investigation.

Side effects, potential complications, and management

Postoperative crusting and discharge

As stated above, oozing and crusting after the procedure are quite common, occurring in almost all patients, especially those with intraoperative serosanguinous discharge or pinpoint bleeding. Minimizing this occurrence starts preoperatively, with advising patients to avoid blood-thinning medications such as non-steroidal anti-inflammatory drugs (NSAIDs) to the extent possible, as well as alcoholic beverages in the few days prior to treatment and in the immediate recovery period. Pinpoint purpura after treatment in a patient taking NSAIDS has also recently been observed [29]. Using treatment depths that match the indication can reduce postoperative discharge as well. Treatments targeted mainly at dyschromic conditions generally need not penetrate so deeply, for example. In the postoperative period, careful gentle cleansing of the skin and dilute vinegar compresses help reduce inflammation, loosen debris, and provide patient comfort. Patients should be cautoned that emollient should be present on the skin at all times until healing is complete.

Local skin reactions

It is fairly common to encounter edema in the immediate postoperative period. For this reason, our standard protocol includes an intramuscular corticosteroid injection prior to treatment. Should this be precluded, superpotent topical corticosteroid application immediately post-treatment should similarly aid in reducing postoperative swelling. Topical or oral corticosteroids can also be used to manage the local irritation and contact dermatitis that can occasionally occur with commonly used emollient preparations, but the practitioner should remain ever suspicious of infection and perform appropriate examination and treatment if needed.

Acneiform eruptions

The development of milia or acneiform lesions after ablative resurfacing is a well-documented phenomenon [1]. While overall seemingly less common with the fractional ablative devices, they do occur. Postponing the use of occlusive emollients until serosanguinous discharge has ceased can reduce their occurrence. When such eruptions do occur, use of a less occlusive emollient such as bland creams or lotions should aid in reducing lesions.

Oral anti-acne antibiotics can also be considered, as topical acne treatment in the immediate postoperative period should generally be avoided but can be undertaken after surface healing is complete.

Post-inflammatory hyperpigmentation

The occurrence of post-inflammatory hyperpigmentation in patients with type III and darker skin is a near certainty. Many patients will have been started on hydroquinone pre-procedure, but whether or not this is the case, it should be implemented post-treatment. Twice-daily application of 4% hydroquinone cream has reduced the severity and duration of hyperpigmentation in patients undergoing treatment in our center. Other topicals can be used adjunctively, such as topical steroids, kojic acid, and tretinoin. A recent report by Tan *et al.* also reported avoidance of hyperpigmentation in seven subjects with type IV–V skin treated with the Lumenis ActiveFX device by treating them on postoperative days 3–14 with 4% hydroquinone in the morning and 0.05% tretinoin in the evenings [30].

Scarring and textural change

While the overall risk of scarring is decidedly less with the fractional ablative devices than with traditional ablative resurfacing lasers, it can occur. Successfully treated incipient early scarring was seen in one patient in an early study [14], and numerous small case series detailing patients who developed scars, primarily from neck treatments [31–33]. Ross and Spencer also recently reported a case of scarring and persistent erythema [34]. Whether using a "stripe" or "stamp" device, it is possible to overlap or perform multiple passes such that near-total ablation is achieved. Given that each laser pulse can be much deeper than traditional ablative pulses, this might have catastrophic potential, as full ablation to dermal levels would lead to certain scarring. In addition to monitoring the technique, and the meticulous aftercare mentioned above, it is especially imperative to caution patients who have their necks treated as to the risk of scarring. These patients should come to the treatment facility wearing clothing that fits loosely around the neck, and should absolutely avoid tight-fitting or "turtleneck" tops and all jewelry. Should early signs of textural change appear, aggressive intervention is warranted. Regular treatment with pulsed dye laser (PDL) and intralesional corticosteroids has proven useful in the authors' experience.

Combination treatments

Many devices are available, but most cannot hope to have access to all! Conversely, as laser surgery becomes more sophisticated, creative combinations have started to appear. Practitioners might suggest that for a patient with generalized dyschromia but only focal rhytides, he or she might benefit from a full-face treatment using a superficial "quasi-fractional" device with wider, shallow ablative characteristics, and localized treatment with a "true fractional" pattern of narrow-but-deep spots. Similarly, a patient with widespread damage that is focally severe, such as in the periorbital area, can be treated in the worst areas with a fully ablative laser, using a fractional ablative device for the rest of the face and/or neck.

Fractional ablative laser treatment has shown the ability to create volumetric tissue reduction and tissue tightening, but there are many factors to take into account in planning appropriate treatment. Much attention has been devoted recently to the multiple factors that contribute to facial aging. The former paradigm that gravity is the main contributor to skin laxity and an "aged" appearance has given way to new discovery that fat atrophy and bone resorption, particularly in the lower face, creates not only skin laxity but also a volume-loss phenomenon [35–37]. This being the case, one would be remiss not to address this loss of volume when undertaking facial rejuvenation. Many techniques exist, such as poly-L-lactic-acid, calcium hydroxylapatite, or autologous fat transfer for large-volume correction of lipoatrophy, as well as agents such as hyaluronic acid, and collagen, for more superficial filling. Combining these techniques with resurfacing can create a more complete aesthetic result.

Conclusions

Fractional ablative resurfacing represents a substantial advancement in the way laser surgeons treat the signs of aging and other dermatologic conditions. In many ways, this is a liberating step, one that allows treatments that are easier to administer, easier for patients to recover from, and less likely to cause adverse effects. In their brief history, these devices have proven quite effective, and, as work continues, the indications for their use will likely broaden, as will their use. While this is certainly an exciting new area of therapy, a word of caution should accompany the excitement. With the return to the use of ablative wavelengths, a return to some of the complications seen with earlier ablative treatments has already been documented, and more cases are likely to be seen. The safety margin with fractional ablative resurfacing is wider than with full ablation, but the careless practitioner can destroy this advantage quite easily. It is the opinion of the authors of this chapter that these lasers are not for the novice laser surgeon, and certainly not for physician extenders, but rather for those with experience with less aggressive devices and treatment protocols.

References

1 Ratner D, Tse Y, Marchell N, Goldman MP, Fitzpatrick RE, Fader DJ. Cutaneous laser resurfacing. *J Am Acad Dermatol* 1999; **41**: 365–89.

2 Dover J, Hruza G. Laser skin resurfacing. *Semin Cutan Med Surg* 1996; **15**: 177–88.

3 Shim E, Tse Y, Velazquez E, Kamino H, Levine V, Ashinoff R. Short-pulse carbon dioxide laser resurfacing in the treatment of rhytides and scars: a clinical and histopathological study. *Dermatol Surg* 1998; **24**: 113–17.

4 Alster TS, Bettencourt MS. Review of cutaneous lasers and their applications. *South Med J* 1998; **91**: 806–14.

5 Flageul G. [The use of an ultrapulse CO_2 laser in the treatment of skin aging]. *Orthod Fr* 1997; **68**: 83–4.

6 Apfelberg DB. Ultrapulse carbon dioxide laser with CPG scanner for full-face resurfacing for rhytids, photoaging, and acne scars. *Plast Reconstr Surg* 1997; **99**: 1817–25.

7 Biesman B. Carbon dioxide laser skin resurfacing. *Semin Ophthalmol* 1998; **13**: 123–35.

8 Fitzpatrick RE, Goldman MP. Advances in carbon dioxide laser surgery. *Clin Dermatol* **13**: 35–47.

9 Alster TS, Lupton JR. An overview of cutaneous laser resurfacing. *Clin Plast Surg* 2001; **28**: 37–52.

10 Alexiades-Armenakas MR, Dover JS, Arndt KA. The spectrum of laser skin resurfacing: nonablative, fractional, and ablative laser resurfacing. *J Am Acad Dermatol* 2008; **58**: 719–37.

11 Sukal SA, Geronemus RG. Fractional photothermolysis. *J Drugs Dermatol* 2008; **7**: 118–22.

12 Hantash BM, Bedi VP, Kapadia B, *et al*. In vivo histological evaluation of a novel ablative fractional resurfacing device. *Lasers Surg Med* 2007; **39**: 96–107.

13 Hantash BM, Bedi VP, Chan KF, Zachary CB. Ex vivo histological characterization of a novel ablative fractional resurfacing device. *Lasers Surg Med* 2007; **39**: 87–95.

14 Rahman Z, MacFalls H, Jiang K, *et al*. Fractional deep dermal ablation induces tissue tightening. *Lasers Surg Med* 2009; **41**: 78–86.

15 Chapas AM, Brightman L, Sukal S, *et al*. Successful treatment of acneiform scarring with CO_2 ablative fractional resurfacing. *Lasers Surg Med* 2008; **40**: 381–6.

16 Walgrave SE, Ortiz AE, MacFalls HT, *et al*. Evaluation of a novel fractional resurfacing device for treatment of acne scarring. *Lasers Surg Med* 2009; **41**: 122–7.

17 Dierickx CC, Khatri KA, Tannous ZS, *et al*. Micro-fractional ablative skin resurfacing with two novel erbium laser systems. *Lasers Surg Med* 2008; **40**: 113–23.

18 Trelles MA, Vélez M, Mordon S. Correlation of histological findings of single session Er:YAG skin fractional resurfacing with various passes and energies and the possible clinical implications. *Lasers Surg Med* 2008; **40**: 171–7.

19 Lapidoth M, Yagima Odo ME, Odo LM. Novel use of erbium:YAG (2940 nm) laser for fractional ablative photothermolysis in the treatment of photodamaged facial skin: a pilot study. *Dermatol Surg* 2008; **34**: 1048–53.

20 Ross EV, Swann M, Soon S, Izadpanah A, Barnette D, Davenport S. Full-face treatments with the 2790 nm erbium:YSGG laser system. *J Drugs Dermatol* 2009; **8**: 248–52.

21 Alster T, Hirsch R. Single-pass CO_2 laser skin resurfacing of light and dark skin: extended experience with 52 patients. *J Cosmet Laser Ther* 2003; **5**: 39–42.

22 Nanni CA, Alster TS. Complications of carbon dioxide laser resurfacing. An evaluation of 500 patients. *Dermatol Surg* 1998; **24**: 315–20.

23 Manuskiatti W, Fitzpatrick RE, Goldman MP, Krejci-Papa N. Prophylactic antibiotics in patients undergoing laser resurfacing of the skin. *J Am Acad Dermatol* 1999; **40**: 77–84.

24 Clementoni MT, Gilardino P, Muti GF, Beretta D, Schianchi R. Non-sequential fractional ultrapulsed CO2 resurfacing of photoaged facial skin: preliminary clinical report. *J Cosmet Laser Ther* 2007; **9**: 218–25.

25 Berlin AL, Hussain M, Phelps R, Goldberg DJ. A prospective study of fractional scanned nonsequential carbon dioxide laser resurfacing: a clinical and histopathologic evaluation. *Dermatol Surg* 2009; **35**: 222–8.

26 Cohen JL, Babcock MJ. Ablative fractionated erbium:YAG laser for the treatment of ice pick alar scars due to neodymium:YAG laser burns. *J Drugs Dermatol* 2009; **8**: 65–7.

27 Waibel J, Beer K. Ablative fractional laser resurfacing for the treatment of a third-degree burn. *J Drugs Dermatol* 2009; **8**: 294–7.

28 Gotkin RH, Sarnoff DS, Cannarozzo G, Sadick NS, Alexiades-Armenakas M. Ablative skin resurfacing with a novel microablative CO_2 laser. *J Drugs Dermatol* 2009; **8**: 138–44.

29 Fife DJ, Zachary CB. Delayed pinpoint purpura after fractionated carbon dioxide treatment in a patient taking ibuprofen in the postoperative period. *Dermatol Surg* 2009; **35**: 553.

30 Tan KL, Kurniawati C, Gold MH. Low risk of postinflammatory hyperpigmentation in skin types 4 and 5 after treatment with fractional CO_2 laser device. *J Drugs Dermatol* 2008; **7**: 774–7.

31 Fife DJ, Fitzpatrick RE, Zachary CB. Complications of fractional CO_2 laser resurfacing: four cases. *Lasers Surg Med* 2009; **41**: 179–84.

32 Biesman BS. Fractional ablative skin resurfacing: complications. *Lasers Surg Med* 2009; **41**: 177–8.

33 Avram MM, Tope WD, Yu T, Szachowicz E, Nelson JS. Hypertrophic scarring of the neck following ablative fractional carbon dioxide laser resurfacing. *Lasers Surg Med* 2009; **41**: 185–8.

34 Ross RB, Spencer J. Scarring and persistent erythema after fractionated ablative CO2 laser resurfacing. *J Drugs Dermatol* 2008; **7**: 1072–3.

35 Ascher B, Coleman S, Alster T, *et al.* Full scope of effect of facial lipoatrophy: a framework of disease understanding. *Dermatol Surg* 2006; **32**: 1058–69.

36 Donofrio L, Weinkle S. The third dimension in facial rejuvenation: a review. *J Cosmet Dermatol* 2006; **5**: 277–83.

37 Donath AS, Glasgold RA, Glasgold MJ. Volume loss versus gravity: new concepts in facial aging. *Curr Opin Otolaryngol Head Neck Surg* 2007; **15**: 238–43.

CHAPTER 4

Non-Surgical Facial Skin Tightening

Jacob Dudelzak[1] and David J. Goldberg[1,2,3]

[1] Skin Laser & Surgery Specialists of New York and New Jersey, USA
[2] Mount Sinai School of Medicine, New York, NY, USA
[3] Sanctuary Medical Aesthetic Center, Boca Raton, FL; USA

Key points

- Non-surgical skin tightening involves bulk heating of dermal collagen
- Initial radiofrequency approaches have now been joined by other light-based technology methods
- Initial treatment algorithms continue to change
- Non-surgical skin tightening approaches continues to improve

---

Introduction

Facial laxity acquired through the normal aging process represents an important cosmetic concern frequently faced by cosmetic surgeons. For years, surgical intervention, including face and neck lifts, was the only means available to address this common problem. However, although this surgical approach provides a rapid and definitive treatment for facial and neck laxity, it is also associated with a host of significant operative risks, ranging from bleeding, ecchymosis, and hematoma formation to incision-site dehiscence and infection. The postoperative healing period is usually lengthy, with significant downtime imposed on the patient. In addition, although usually highly effective, a surgical approach to the treatment of facial and neck laxity may impart an exaggerated artificial appearance. And, as the individual continues to age following the face- or neck-lifting procedure and the normal distribution of subcutaneous fat continues to shift, a cosmetically undesirable appearance of pronounced superolateral pulling may develop. These drawbacks to the surgical approach have led many patients in search of less aggressive non-invasive or minimally invasive procedures with shorter downtime and cosmetic results that, although overall more subtle, yet bestow upon an individual a less overt and more "natural" and gradual improvement.

Facial Resurfacing, 1st edition. Edited by David J. Goldberg. © 2010 Blackwell Publishing.

As the field of minimally invasive cosmetic dermatology continues to expand, new innovative techniques and technologies are emerging that may provide relatively safer and less morbid solutions, associated with shorter downtime, compared with the more aggressive and invasive surgical techniques.

Laser and light-based technology

Some of the earlier non-surgical methods developed for the treatment of facial laxity and rhytides included chemical peels, dermabrasion, and ablative laser resurfacing. Laser resurfacing, typically employing an ablative carbon dioxide (CO_2) or an erbium:yttrium–aluminum–garnet (Er:YAG) technology, was successful in providing means for tissue tightening by producing thermal injury within the dermal collagen, leading to immediate collagen contraction and subsequent collagen remodeling through a wound healing process.

The process by which ablative laser systems elicit collagen changes within the dermis relies on the principle of selective photothermolysis, whereby optical energy emitted by the laser is absorbed by a target chromophore within the treated tissue, in this case water, and is subsequently dissipated within the surrounding tissue as generated heat. However, given the ubiquity of the water chromophore within the various cutaneous levels, the heat generated by this process produces thermal injury non-specifically within the skin that often leads to epidermal disruption and considerable risk of scarring [1–3].

Other limitations of laser and light-based systems in eliciting significant deep dermal and subcutaneous tissue tightening stem from the considerable attenuation of optic energy as it passes through the treated skin as a result of light scattering and absorption by epidermal melanin. Consequently, the emission of greater fluences by a light-based system is often necessary to deliver optic energies high enough to elicit meaningful changes on the deep dermal and subcuticular collagen. This, in turn, increases the likelihood of producing excessive tissue thermal injury, including epidermal ablation, and consequently leads to treatment-associated pain and an increased risk of side effects, including persistent erythema, post-inflammatory pigmentary alteration, and scarring, as well as a prolonged postoperative healing period. Furthermore, this approach may be associated with a greater risk of treatment-associated side effects in patients with darker complexion or Asian skin type [1–3].

Non-ablative tissue tightening has been the focus within the field of facial aesthetics in the past several years. Compared with earlier CO_2 resurfacing techniques, this new approach, if used properly, provides patients with an alternative in achieving skin tightening of the face and neck regions with minimal to no downtime and significantly reduced risk of complications [1–3].

Radiofrequency technology

Radiofrequency (RF) technology is neither very new nor limited to the field of aesthetic surgery. RF devices have been used successfully in many fields of medicine for various indications, including for electrocoagulation and electrodessication, as well as in corneal, vascular, orthopedic, and cardiac surgery. Examples of such applications include the treatment of ectopic arrhythmogenic foci within the heart, ablation of hepatic and renal tumors, and treatment of intracranial neurofibromas in patients afflicted by neurofibromatosis [4–9].

The mechanism of all RF devices is similar to the light and laser-based systems in that it relies on the production of heat within the treated tissue that effects changes in collagen. However, unlike a light-based device, which relies on the principle of selective photothermolysis, the heat energy generated by an RF system is produced according to Ohm's law [1,2,10].

Ohm's law states that the energy delivered is directly proportional to the product of the square of the current, the impedance, and the time of application. Each RF device establishes an electromagnetic field within the treated tissue, resulting in the movement of charged particles directed from one pole or electrode to the other. This movement of charged particles is termed a current. All tissues possess an intrinsic property of impedance, or its resistance to the movement of charged particles within the electromagnetic field. Physical and electrical properties of the tissue determine the degree of impedance it provides. For instance, the impedance of subcutaneous fat and bone is considerably higher than the impedance of muscle and dermis. Thus, current passing through tissues of higher impedance, such as the subcutaneous fat and bone, will generate a greater amount of heat energy than that flowing through lower-impedance tissues, such as muscle and dermis. Finally, the length of time the current is applied determines the amount of energy that will be generated. Thus, unlike the optical-based devices, the process by which RF devices generate heat is not chromophore-dependent, but rather is a function of the current, the tissue impedance, and the time of application [10].

The tissue tightening elicited by RF devices has two phases, immediate and delayed. The immediate skin tightening observed clinically following RF treatment occurs as a result of collagen contraction response to thermal injury. As a result of volumetric heating, hydrogen bonds within the collagen triple helix are broken, resulting in the morphologic changes of the collagen fibrils, or denaturation, from a crystalline to an amorphous form. These changes, evidenced by collagen contraction, are seen on ultra-structural examination via transmission electron microscopy within the mid to deep dermis. Collagen fibril thickening and shortening resulting from this process impart greater elastic properties to the molecule, leading to contraction and tissue tightening. In addition to dermal collagen contraction, skin tightening observed in the immediate post-treatment period also results from heat-mediated contraction of the subcutaneous fibrous septae [11,12].

The target temperature at which dermal collagen denaturation occurs ranges from 58 to 75 °C. Above these temperatures, liquefaction of collagen and other dermal proteins takes place, leading to a loss of any significant collagen elasticity, and therefore resulting in the absence of a tissue-tightening response [13].

The immediate tissue tightening seen in response to RF treatment is followed by a gradual skin tightening occurring over several weeks to 4–6 months, reflecting new collagen synthesis and collagen remodeling during a process of delayed wound healing. Collagen remodeling has been previously documented by immunohistochemical studies of treated skin, showing upregulation of type I collagen, type III procollagen, tropoelastin, matrix metalloproteinases, and cytokines. The effects on collagen have also been observed via transmission electron microscopy [11,14].

In contrast to the laser and light-based systems, in which selective photothermolysis requires a target chromophore, the energy delivered by RF devices is chromophore-independent, and no light scattering occurs in the process. The greater depth of penetration by the electric energy of RF systems allows collagen contraction and remodeling to occur within the deep reticular dermis and subcutaneous tissue, which is often necessary to achieve clinically significant tissue tightening. Furthermore, lower fluences may be utilized to deliver adequate heating to deep dermal collagen to elicit contraction and remodeling. In addition, the lack of absorption by epidermal melanin allows RF modalities to be used in relative safety in the treatment of facial and neck laxity in patients with darker skin types [12].

Several types of radiofrequency devices have been developed over the last 10 years. Their emitted energy ranges in frequency from 3 kHz to 300 MHz. Some deliver monopolar RF as a current between a single electrode and a dispersive electrode, also called the grounding plate. Others produce a bipolar RF current traveling between two points on the tip of the probe. A grounding plate is not used in this system, and no current passes through the body, except within the treated area between the two electrodes. Two methods of delivery of the bipolar RF energy exist: parallel, in which the RF current passes directly through the treated skin suctioned into the field between two parallel electrodes; and linear, in which the RF current arcs through the treated skin from one electrode to another arranged perpendicularly to the skin surface. Yet another method employs unipolar RF electromagnetic radiation (EMR) [3].

One of the advantages of the monopolar RF system is the greater depth of penetration attained by the RF energy, compared to that delivered by the bipolar system, in which the treatment field is confined to the area between the two treating electrodes. The depth of current penetration in a bipolar system can be estimated as half the distance separating the two electrodes. Thus, the monopolar system is more likely to produce changes within the deep dermis and the subcutaneous tissue. On the other hand, given these properties, the bipolar system provides for a more controlled delivery of energy and may also be associated with less treatment-associated discomfort and potential for adverse side effects [1,3].

Available systems and treatment approaches

Currently available technologies employing the RF method of tissue tightening include the ThermaCool® monopolar RF device (Thermage, Hayward, CA), the Aluma® bipolar RF system with FACES® technology (Lumenis Inc., Santa Clara, CA), the ST ReFirme® linear bipolar RF in combination with red light (Syneron, Yokneam, Israel), the Polaris® linear bipolar RF device in combination with diode laser (Syneron, Yokneam, Israel), the Aurora® linear bipolar RF device in combination with diode laser and intense pulsed light (Syneron, Yokneam, Israel), and the Accent® device with bipolar RF and unipolar EMR handpieces (Alma Lasers, Caesarea, Israel) (Fig. 4.1).

Monopolar RF systems
The first radiofrequency device introduced in the United States was the ThermaCool TC monopolar RF (Figs. 4.2–4.4), first approved by the US Food and Drug Administration for non-invasive treatment of facial rhytides. The device has since been used successfully in the treatment of facial laxity, from jowl lifting and definition of the cervicomental angle, to amelioration of the nasolabial folds, to brow lifting on the order of 1–4 mm, to tightening of the upper eyelid skin and decrease in the periorbital rhytides. Non-facial tightening applications of the ThermaCool system include treatment of facial acne vulgaris and reduction in the appearance of pores [1,12–24].

The device utilizes a high-frequency generator producing a 330 watt powered, 6 MHz monopolar electrical current rapidly alternating at 6 million times per second, establishing an electrical field and providing volumetric tissue heating to a depth of 3–6 mm. Epidermal cooling before, during, and after RF current delivery is achieved using a cryogen spray delivered

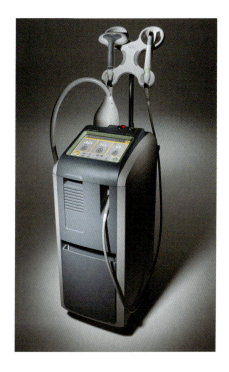

Figure 4.1 Accent radiofrequency device containing both a unipolar and a bipolar handpiece (Alma Lasers, Caesarea, Israel).

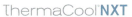

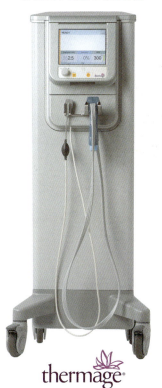

Figure 4.2 ThermaCool monopolar radiofrequency device (Thermage, Haywood, CA). Reproduced with the permission of Solta Medical.

ThermaCool®**NXT**

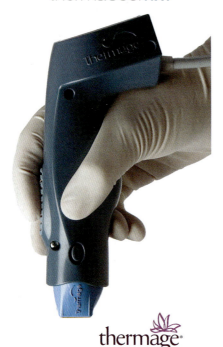

Figure 4.3 ThermaCool treatment handpiece with a 1 cm² fast tip. Reproduced with the permission of Solta Medical.

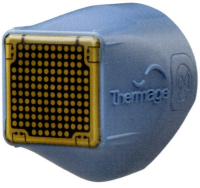

Thermage Face Tip: 3.0

Figure 4.4 ThermaCool 3.0 cm treatment tip. Reproduced with the permission of Solta Medical.

through the treatment tip membrane. Surface cooling establishes a reverse thermal gradient, which focuses thermal heat deposition deeper within the dermis and away from the surface where excessive heat could produce epidermal damage. The computer-controlled sensors within the treatment tip constantly monitor and provide the system with data on the delivered energy, temperature, and pressure. Pressure and temperature sensors at each corner of the treatment tip ensure that the treatment cycle is aborted if the system detects incomplete contact with the treatment site or if the surface temperature exceeds a set threshold, providing an important safeguard [11,12].

A dispersive electrode is placed on the body far removed from the target tissue area, typically on the back, which functions to direct and absorb the monopolar current emanating from the active electrode, or probe, located within the treatment tip [1].

The treatment tip measures both local and bulk tissue impedance and provides the system with feedback on the total. Local tissue impedance is a measure of the resistance to the absorption of energy in the tissue being treated, while bulk impedance is that encountered by the current in remote non-heated tissue on the way to the dispersive electrode. It is thought that the bulk impedance is the primary parameter affecting combined impedance. In providing a consistent energy delivery, the ThermaCool TC device is programmed to increase the delivered current in response to lowered impedance above 120 ohms [25].

Several treatment tips have been developed, including the 0.25 cm^2, 1 cm^2, 1.5 cm^2, and 3 cm^2, with smaller tips allowing precise treatment in periorbital areas while larger tips permit an efficient management of laxity over larger surface areas, such as the abdomen, arms, and thighs. Given that the system utilizes a monopolar RF energy delivery, a grounding pad is attached to the patient prior to the therapy session far removed from the treatment area. An ink grid developed by the manufacturer is imprinted on the treatment area, consisting of squares corresponding to an area slightly smaller than the treatment tip, which allows for monitoring of the areas treated, ensuring complete coverage and preventing unnecessary overlap. A coupling fluid placed on the patient's skin provides for appropriate flow of RF energy through a coupling membrane, leading to volumetric tissue heating [1].

The approach to treatment of facial skin laxity with the monopolar RF device has undergone significant modification over the past several years. Initially, the treatment was given as a single pass over the entire target area, such as the face, using relatively high fluences. Preoperative topical anesthetic preparations, as well as nerve blocks, were commonly administered in order to alleviate the often significant treatment-associated patient discomfort. This single-pass high-fluence approach was subsequently overtaken in popularity by a novel lower-fluence, multiple-pass algorithm.

This new technique also emphasizes the role that patient feedback on pain sensation provides in selecting an appropriate energy level. The proponents of this approach argue that by selecting a treatment fluence within a moderate range, rather than at the highest level of the individual's pain scale, the clinician would not only provide a more comfortable treatment to the patient, but also would avoid inflicting excessive heat injury to the treated tissue, thus decreasing the risk of potential complications such as scarring and post-inflammatory pigmentary changes. Still others advocate against the use of topical anesthetic agents or nerve blocks during treatment, as they not only do not significantly reduce the type of pain associated with the deep dermal heating produced by the RF devices, but also preclude the appropriate assessment of the pain level by the patient, whose feedback on it is considered vital in the selection of the appropriate energy density [18].

As will be discussed later in greater detail, multiple studies have been conducted to determine the efficacy and safety of the low-fluence, multiple-pass RF approach, comparing the results to those of earlier studies with the high-fluence, single-pass technique. The findings suggest that the newer technique produces a greater clinical improvement in facial skin laxity, while having a safer side-effect profile, better patient tolerability, and greater overall patient satisfaction.

Generally, the entire area is first treated with two passes, followed by additional passes over the areas of problematic laxity, particularly the jowls, the submental region, and the areas of the cheeks adjoining the nasolabial folds, performed in the direction of the treatment vectors. The additional passes are also thought to provide greater heating to the deeper subcutaneous fibrous septae, to effect contraction at this layer in addition to that achieved within the dermis [1].

The delivered fluences should be tailored to the individual patient's pain threshold. The end-point for treatment is considered to be visible tissue tightening and erythema. Lower fluences are generally selected when treating thinner skin areas, such as the forehead and neck, areas overlying the supraorbital, infraorbital, and greater auricular nerves, as well as over the temporal and malar regions. The number of pulses delivered during a treatment session varies based upon the facial region being treated, from 40–80 in the periorbital areas to 600 for a full-face treatment [15–19].

Side effects reported in studies involving monopolar radiofrequency treatment include transient erythema and edema, generally resolving within 1–2 days following treatment. The occurrence of persistent edema that resolved with a course of oral steroid treatment has been reported. Reports of small superificial burns are most commonly associated with incomplete skin contact with the treatment tip or premature removal of the tip from the skin surface precluding post-pulse cooling. Transient skin numbness, most commonly in the sensory distribution of the greater auricular nerve, has also been described. Temporary skin ridging in the neck overlying the platysma muscle has been linked to higher utilized fluences. Reports of tissue irregularity resulting from excessive tissue heating have also been published [10–24].

Bipolar RF systems

The Aluma bipolar RF device introduced by Lumenis Inc. employs the "Functional Aspiration Controlled by Electrothermal Stimulation" (FACES) technology. Following contact of the two treatment electrodes with the skin surface, this system generates a vacuum that elevates a flap of target skin into the space between the electrodes, thus allowing for a greater depth of bipolar RF energy penetration. The device may be operated using the 3 mm × 18 mm or the 6 mm × 25 mm treatment tips [26].

Infrared systems

The Titan® infrared device (Cutera Inc., Brisbane, CA, USA; Fig. 4.5) has recently been introduced in the field of non-surgical skin tightening. The device is a non-coherent, selectively filtered infrared lamp light source. The emitted 1100–1800 nm energy is filtered at 1400–1500 nm, and delivered with multisecond-long pulses (up to 8.1 s), with available spot sizes of 1.5 cm × 1 cm and 3 cm × 1 cm. The 1400–1500 nm attenuation is necessary given the strong water absorption in this wavelength range, which could result in excessive heating. Epidermal pre-, parallel-, and post-cooling are provided by a temperature-regulated sapphire window in contact with the skin surface. Fluences of up to 50 J/cm^2 may be attained [27,28].

The mechanism of action in producing dermal heating and consequent thermal collagen injury necessary to initiate the collagen remodeling process is the targeted heating by this long-wavelength device of its water chromophore. In contrast to flashlamp-based devices, which emit at shorter wavelengths, usually in the visible light range, and are pulsed at shorter millisecond pulses, this infrared broadband lamp-based device delivers

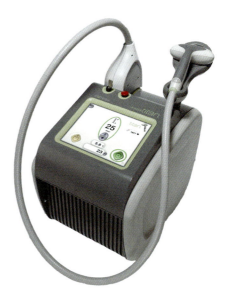

Figure 4.5 Titan infrared device (Cutera Inc., Brisbane, CA, USA).

higher-wavelength multisecond pulses that are designed to provide a more uniform dermal heating over a broad treatment area [27,28].

This new device also differs from other infrared devices in its relatively lower level of water absorption, longer multisecond, rather than millisecond, pulse durations, and a larger spot size, all intended to elicit deeper and more gradual tissue heating. It is estimated that the depth of heat penetration of this device is 1–2 mm (and up to 5 mm), which targets the collagen within the reticular dermis [27,28].

Proponents of this device argue that given that the collagen contraction phenomenon is a function of both the exposure time and the delivered temperature, the longer multisecond pulse delivery approach allows collagen contraction to occur at lower target heating temperatures of 60–65 °C due to the increased exposure time, thus allowing for lower treatment fluences to be used. In contrast, millisecond pulse duration devices deliver short exposure with high fluences to elicit collagen contraction at target temperature of 85 °C, which may increase the risk of treatment-associated side effects and produce greater pain [29].

Protective eyewear is a mandatory precaution for the patient as well as the treating physician. As with the monopolar radiofrequency device, the treatment is undertaken in several passes. Two passes are generally performed over the entire treatment area, followed by additional passes over the areas of pronounced laxity. Between 200 and 250 pulses with fluences of 30 J/cm^2 have been utilized successfully over most of the face, with lower fluences of 25 J/cm^2 employed over the thin-skin areas or bony prominences, such as the forehead and temples. Ensuring a complete skin contact with the cool sapphire crystal tip is of paramount importance in order to avoid excessive heating and epidermal ablation. Side effects of treatment reported in studies range from the most common small superficial burns to the rare third-degree burns, usually resulting from improper technique or excessive energy delivery [1,28,29].

Electro-optical synergy

A recently introduced concept of electro-optical synergy (ELOS), employed by several new systems, combines light energy in the form of laser, such as the diode laser, intense pulsed light, or a broadband infrared light, together with radiofrequency energy, to impart changes in dermal collagen and effect skin tightening. The proponents of these systems postulate that the advantage of this combined method of therapy stems from the synergistic effects that the radiofrequency and light energies provide in producing collagen contraction and stimulating collagen remodeling, while at the same time allowing for lower energies to be delivered by the combined system, compared with either RF or light modality alone. The decrease in the utilized energy densities would, in turn, minimize the potential for treatment-associated adverse effects and reduce patient discomfort during therapy [30].

One example of such a system is the Aurora SR, which combines bipolar radiofrequency energy of up to 25 J/cm^3, delivered to a depth of 4 mm, with intense pulsed light, emitted in the 400–980 nm, 580–980 nm, and 680–980 nm ranges. In the case of this modality, the optical energy supplied by the intense pulsed light preheats the treated tissue according to the principle of chromophore-dependent selective photothermolysis. The resulting temperature gradient established between the selectively heated dermal tissue and its surroundings, augmented by the epidermal cooling provided by the device, sets up an impedance gradient, with the heated tissues having a lower impedance compared to the cooler surrounding and overlying skin. This impedance gradient provides for a directed flow of RF energy to the IPL pre-heated dermis, with relative sparing of the overlying epidermis and the surrounding skin.

Another system introduced by Syneron that is based on the principle of electro-optical synergy is the Polaris® WR. This system combines a 900 nm diode laser with a bipolar RF energy device, delivering 10–50 J/cm^2 of optical fluences and 10–100 J/cm^3 of RF energies.

New systems

Investigation is currently under way involving a novel 1310 nm diode laser system (Candela Corporation, Wayland, MA) for non-ablative skin tightening. The device allows the operator control of the pulse duration and surface cooling in order to localize the heating at a particular depth within the dermis. Cooling is provided by a cold sapphire plate. Compared with the broadband infrared Titan device, which emits a non-coherent light consisting of a range of wavelengths of various absorption and depths of penetration, the 1310 nm diode laser emits a coherent single-wavelength light with predictable depth of penetration. Furthermore, unlike the Titan device, in which the system automatically determines the pulse duration based on selected fluence, the operator of this new laser system can choose a pulse duration to help localize the heating to within a particular layer within the skin, providing either more superficial or deeper heating.

Objective outcome measures: skin laxity

The ever-growing number of systems introduced into the field of non-ablative skin tightening has prompted some to develop methods of objective measurement of the degree of skin laxity observed in a given patient. This measurement may be ascertained in subjects at baseline and following treatment, proving a reliable and reproducible method that may be used by investigators to assess improvement attained after a given treatment modality. It is hoped that such standardized system of measuring and characterizing skin laxity would lead to a decrease in the inter-observer variability intrinsic to subjective analysis.

One such approach is the Leal laxity classification system. This method allows an investigator to characterize the type, as well as the degree, of laxity. In assessing a subject, four regions of the face are delineated. The upper face is defined as that facial region located superior to the pupillary line; the middle face is bordered superiorly on the pupillary line and inferiorly on the oral commissure; the lower face extends from the oral commissure to the jawline; and the upper neck is defined as the submandibular region superior to the thyroid cartilage. Each region receives individual evaluation in terms of the type and the degree of laxity.

Three types of laxity are defined in the Leal classification. Type A skin is characterized by superficial skin laxity. Type B skin possesses laxity limited to the deeper subcutaneous tissues. Finally, type AB skin is defined as having both a cutaneous and subcutaneous laxity. The "pinch test" is commonly employed to establish the type of laxity a given subject displays. The degree of laxity is measured on a 0–5 scale, with 0 defined as no laxity and 5 defined as extreme laxity. The efficacy of a given non-ablative skin tightening system may be then be quantified by observing the number of treated subjects who experience a decrease on this 6-point scale toward 0 and a change in the type of laxity from type B to type A, or from type AB to either type A or type B.

Figures 4.6 to 4.20 show examples of the results achieved in treating skin laxity with RF and infrared devices.

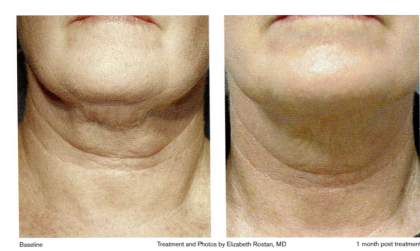

Baseline   Treatment and Photos by Elizabeth Rostan, MD   1 month post treatment

Figure 4.6 Improvement in the neck laxity with decrease in the submental fat following treatment with the monopolar RF ThermaCool device: (left) before treatment; (right) 1 month after treatment.

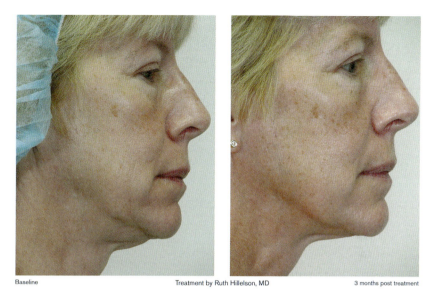

Baseline   Treatment by Ruth Hillelson, MD   3 months post treatment

Figure 4.7 Decrease in lower facial laxity and greater definition of the cervicomandibular angle definition following treatment with the monopolar RF ThermaCool device: (left) before treatment; (right) 3 months after treatment.

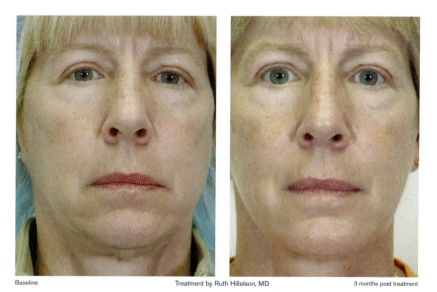

Baseline   Treatment by Ruth Hillelson, MD   3 months post treatment

Figure 4.8 Decrease in lower facial and jowl laxity following treatment with the monopolar RF ThermaCool device: (left) before treatment; (right) 3 months after treatment.

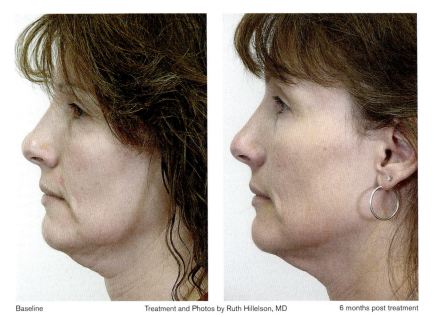

Baseline   Treatment and Photos by Ruth Hillelson, MD   6 months post treatment

Figure 4.9 Decrease in lower facial and jowl laxity, as well as improved definition of the cervicomandibular angle following treatment with the monopolar RF ThermaCool device: (left) before treatment; (right) 6 months after treatment.

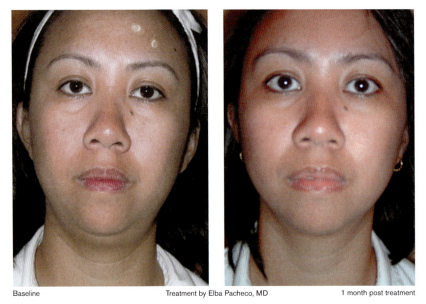

Baseline   Treatment by Elba Pacheco, MD   1 month post treatment

Figure 4.10 Decrease in submental skin laxity following treatment with the monopolar RF ThermaCool device: (left) before treatment; (right) 1 month after treatment.

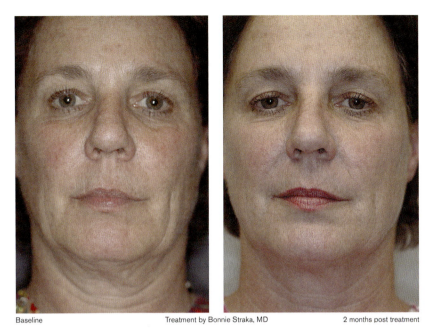

Baseline   Treatment by Bonnie Straka, MD   2 months post treatment

Figure 4.11 Softening of the nasolabial folds and decrease in the lower facial and neck laxity following treatment with the monopolar RF ThermaCool device: (left) before treatment; (right) 2 months after treatment.

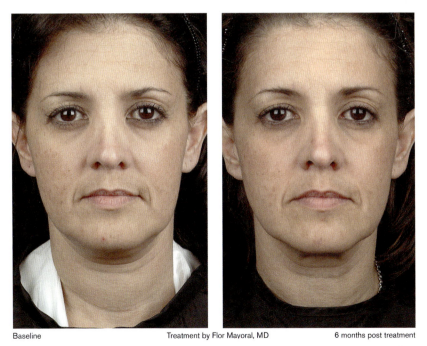

Baseline   Treatment by Flor Mayoral, MD   6 months post treatment

Figure 4.12 Submental tightening in a patient following treatment with the monopolar RF ThermaCool device: (left) before treatment; (right) 6 months after treatment.

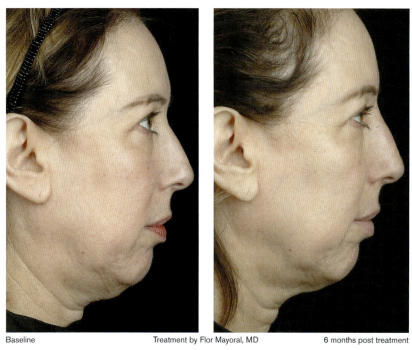

Baseline   Treatment by Flor Mayoral, MD   6 months post treatment

Figure 4.13 Decrease in jowl and neck laxity following treatment with the monopolar RF ThermaCool device: (left) before treatment; (right) 6 months after treatment.

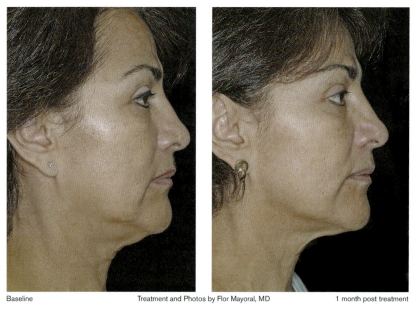

Baseline   Treatment and Photos by Flor Mayoral, MD   1 month post treatment

Figure 4.14 Lower facial tightening and improvement of the cervicomandibular angle in a patient following monopolar RF ThermaCool device: (left) before treatment; (right) 1 month after treatment.

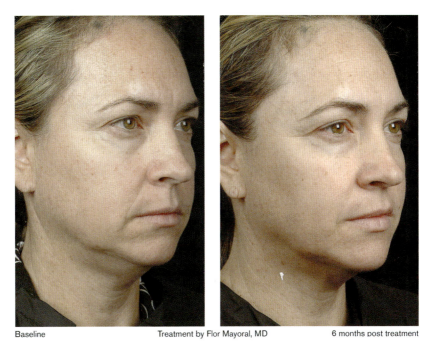

Baseline   Treatment by Flor Mayoral, MD   6 months post treatment

Figure 4.15 Softening of the nasolabial fold lines and tightening of the lower face following monopolar RF ThermaCool device: (left) before treatment; (right) 6 months after treatment.

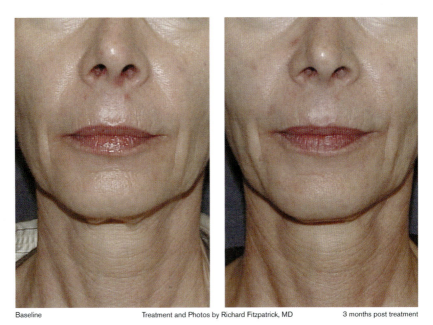

Baseline   Treatment and Photos by Richard Fitzpatrick, MD   3 months post treatment

Figure 4.16 Softening of the nasolabial fold lines and decrease in lower facial laxity following monopolar RF ThermaCool device: (left) before treatment; (right) 3 months after treatment.

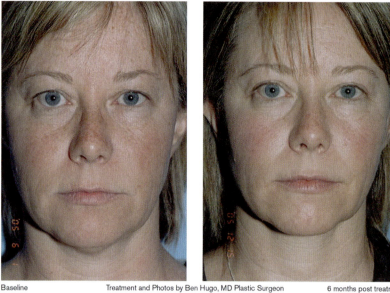

Baseline   Treatment and Photos by Ben Hugo, MD Plastic Surgeon   6 months post treatment

Figure 4.17 Improvement of lower facial tissue irregularities and decrease in jowl laxity following monopolar RF ThermaCool device: (left) before treatment; (right) 3 months after treatment.

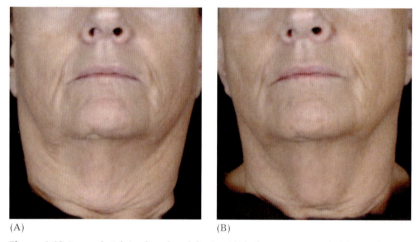

(A)   (B)

Figure 4.18 Lower facial, jowl, and neck laxity: (A) before treatment; (B) 3 months after treatment with Titan infrared device.

Clinical studies

A number of significant clinical studies have been undertaken in the past several years, introducing the various non-ablative tightening devices to the community, establishing the safety of the devices, measuring the degree

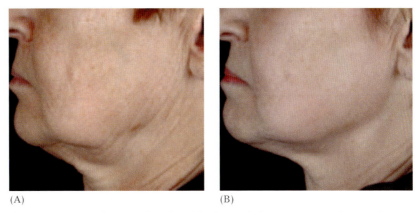

(A)   (B)

Figure 4.19 Lower facial, jowl, and neck laxity: (A) before treatment; (B) 3 months after treatment with Titan infrared device.

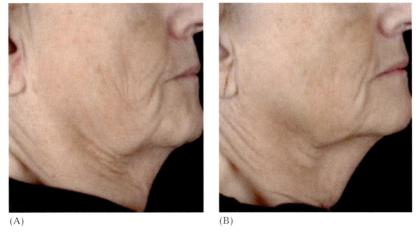

(A)   (B)

Figure 4.20 Lower facial, jowl, and neck laxity: (A) before treatment; (B) 3 months after treatment with Titan infrared device.

of improvement attained by patients treated using these techniques, and finally refining the treatment parameters to optimize efficacy, decrease side effects, and improve patient satisfaction.

One of the first large-scale studies conducted on the use of monopolar radiofrequency device was performed by Fitzpatrick and colleagues in 2003. The study aimed to evaluate the utility of this device in providing periorbital tissue tightening. Eighty-six patients were enrolled in the study, with a mean age of 54 and Fitzpatrick skin types I–IV (primarily type II). On average, the subjects had a Fitzpatrick wrinkle classification system score of 4.7 on a scale of 1–9. Each patient underwent a single monopolar RF treatment using the ThermaCool TC device. The number of treatment pulses ranged from 23 to 114 (average 68). The energy setting ranged from 11 to

21 (average 16), corresponding to 58–140 J/cm^2 delivered energy density. All patients received treatment using the 1 cm^2 treatment tip, with two subjects receiving additional pulses with the 0.25 cm^2 tip. Prior to RF treatment, topical 5% lidocaine was applied for 45 minutes. Twenty-two patients also received nerve blocks [23].

At 6-month follow-up visit, 83.2% of patients were noted by independent and blinded photograph reviewers to have experienced an improvement in the Fitzpatrick wrinkle classification system score, 14.3% of patients experienced no change, and 2.5% of patients worsened. Of the patients experiencing improvement in the wrinkle score, 64.6% improved by 1 point, 31.3% by 2 points, and 4% by 3 or more points. Investigator-assigned wrinkle score at a 6-month follow-up visit showed that 28.9% of patients experienced improvement in the wrinkle score, 63.9% showed no change, and 7.2% worsened. Of note, the percentage of patients showing improvement in the wrinkle score increased from 25% at 2 months to 28.9% at 6 months. Computer-assisted measurement of the eyebrow lift occurring as a result of treatment showed elevation above the 0.5 mm minimum detectable threshold in 61.5% of patients at the 6-month follow-up visit. The eyebrows lifted on average by 1.49 mm on the right and by 1.3 mm on the left side. Patient satisfaction surveys showed that 38% of subjects were satisfied and 12% very satisfied with the results. Increase in tightness was noted by 45% of patients. Improvement in appearance was reported by 49% of subjects. Treatment-associated discomfort was rated by the patients as mild in 40% of treatments on the right and 45% on the left side, moderate in 38% on the right and 35% on the left, severe in 9% on the right and 13% on the left, and intolerable in 1% on the right and 3% on the left [23].

Several types of treatment-associated side effects were reported in the study. These included immediate erythema in 36% of patients, occurring within 72 hours in 16.7%; immediate edema in 13.9% of patients, occurring within 72 hours in 6.4%. Persistent erythema was noted at the 1-month follow-up visit in 3.9% of patients. Scabbing was noted in 7.7% of patients in the initial post-treatment visits, decreasing to 1.4% at 2 months. Twenty-one incidences of second-degree burns were reported in the study, 15 superficial and six deep. This corresponds to a burn risk of 0.36% per application. Of the patients developing burns, three experienced residual scarring, one a focal textural change, and in one scarring resolved within 6 months. No third-degree burns were reported in the study. Three patients experienced forehead bruising resolving within 3–4 weeks. Two subjects who received nerve blocks developed dysesthesia thought to be related to the anesthesia. Urticarial reaction within the treatment area was noted in one patient who was anesthetized with a nerve block and was treated at higher fluences. Headaches developed by three patients were not attributed to therapy [23].

Another 2003 study conducted by Ruiz-Esparza and Gomez involved 15 female patients, ages 41–68, having Fitzpatrick skin types II–V. One-hour application of the ELA-Max 4% lidocaine preparation (Ferndale Laboratories Inc., Ferndale, MI) was used for topical anesthesia prior to the procedure. The Thermage system was utilized in the study to treat a 2.5 cm × 4.5 cm area of the preauricular cheek using a single-pass technique. Five patients were treated using the 0.25 cm² bipolar electrode. Eight were treated with a "window frame" bipolar electrode. These two groups were treated using current settings of 0.201–0.395 ohms. Two patients were treated with the 1 cm² monopolar electrode at 52 J/cm² of fluence [24].

The authors noted a gradual improvement in most patients beginning at 12 weeks following treatment, with the exception of one subject who experienced tightening 1 week post-procedure. Investigator assessment showed a greater than 50% improvement in the softening of the nasolabial folds in 50% of treated subjects. A greater than 50% improvement in cheek tightening was observed in 60% of patients. A greater than 50% improvement in the marionette lines was noted in over 65% of patients. Improvement of the mandibular edge was less prevalent, with only 27% of patients experiencing an over 50% improvement. One subject with a considerable subcutaneous fat component to the cheeks did not respond to therapy. Side effects reported in the study included a superficial burn on the temple of one patient, resulting in a scar that resolved in 3 months with the aid of microdermabrasion. All patients tolerated treatment well. No postoperative swelling, ecchymosis, or pain was reported in the study [24].

In a 2005 study by Kushikata *et al.*, the investigators evaluated the non-ablative monopolar RF device (ThermaCool TC) for treatment of facial laxity in 85 Japanese females aged 31–68 (mean 52.3) years. A 5% lidocaine topical anesthetic cream (ELA-Max) was applied to the treatment area for 50–60 minutes. The treatment with the monopolar RF device was undertaken over the cheeks and jowls using fluences of 74–124 J/cm² (corresponding to treatment levels of 12–15), performed in a single pass, on average 68 pulses on each cheek. Treatment fluences were set based on the patient's maximum tolerance level [21].

At 3-month follow-up, investigators noted at least a 10% improvement in skin laxity of jowls in 78% of patients, of marionette lines in 69.5% of patients, and of nasolabial folds in 73.8% of patients. This improved further to 89% for jowls, 89% for marionette lines, and 83.8% for nasolabial folds at the 6-month follow-up visit. On the other hand, patient satisfaction declined from 79.3% for jowls, 67.1% for marionette lines, and 76.3% for nasolabial folds at 3 months, to 76.8% for jowls, 63.4% for marionette lines, and 72.5% for nasolabial folds. Treatment side effects reported in the study consisted of post-treatment edema in three patients, a burn in one patient, a blister in one patient, and post-inflammatory hyperpigmentation in two patients. Both the burn and the blister formation were evident within the hour of RF treatment. On the other hand, pigment alteration changes appeared at 1 month following the treatment session. In patients experiencing burn and blister formation, both healed without pigmentary changes. However, the patients experiencing delayed hyperpigmentation required 3 months for resolution, albeit without necessitating therapy [21].

Another 2005 study conducted by Finzi and Spangler evaluated the multi-pass vector technique (mpave) for non-ablative radiofrequency skin tightening of face and neck. Twenty-five patients with Fitzpatrick skin types I–V with mild to severe facial and neck laxity were enrolled in the study. A single treatment session with the monopolar RF ThermaCool TC device was undertaken by each patient [31].

Prior to the procedure the direction of each desired tissue tightening vector was ascertained by gently pulling the target skin. Most patients exhibited two major vectors. The inferior jaw and neck vector was directed at 60° inferior to the horizontal line connecting the root of the ear helix and the nose. The mid-face vector was directed at 30° inferior to the same horizontal line. In addition to applying the treatment grid to the entire face, these vectors were also marked on the skin in a multi-teardrop configuration to avoid pronounced contrast between these areas targeted for multi-pass therapy and the rest of the face undergoing a single-pass treatment. Each smaller teardrop zone was treated with a greater number of passes, compared to the larger teardrop zone, the smallest teardrop receiving five passes. Fluence selection was based on the patient's pain level, and ranged from 73 to 85 J/cm^2. Treatment was undertaken using the 1 cm^2 fast tip. Two mid-facial rows of pulses were performed to effect treatment of the pronounced nasolabial folds [31].

The appropriate upper facial vector was assessed to allow eyebrow lifting, with some patients requiring a uniform brow lift while others needed a more lateral brow elevation. For lateral brow lift, three columns of pulses were placed superior to the lateral eyebrow border, whereas three columns of pulses placed uniformly superior to the entire eyebrow were performed if a general eyebrow lift was desired. Care was taken to avoid pulses beyond the temporal fusion line in order to decrease the risk of fat atrophy. Eyebrow lift fluences ranged from 73 to 85 J/cm^2 [31].

The treatment of the neck was preceded by delineating the neck into two parts: the submental region and the lateral neck areas. The lateral neck areas were treated at fluences of 68–85 J/cm^2 with three passes of 2–4 inframandibular rows of pulses. The submental region was treated with three passes at 68–85 J/cm^2, with an additional two stacked passes performed over areas of excess subcutaneous fat at an energy density of 62 J/cm^2 [31].

Three months after the treatment session, marked (76–100%) clinical improvement in facial and neck laxity was noted in 4% of patients;

excellent (51–75%) improvement in 20% of patients; moderate (26–50%) improvement in 56% of patients; and mild (1–25%) improvement in 16% of patients. Thus, 96% of patients were able to attain some clinical response with the mpave technique. In most patients, maximum clinical improvement was attained at 12 weeks following treatment. One patient, 68 years of age, showed no improvement. Patients treated with pulse stacking in the submental region experienced fat reduction after treatment. Side effects reported in the study included bruising, periorbital edema lasting up to 1 week in two patients, and transient submental dysesthesia resolving within 6 weeks in two patients. No burns, pigmentary alteration, or scarring was reported [31].

In 2005, Lack *et al.* examined the relationship of energy settings and impedance in various anatomic areas treated with a monopolar radiofrequency device, ThermaCool TC. Four patients were enrolled in the study, ages 23–52. Each patient was treated with a single pulse using the 1 cm^2 tip at a treatment setting of 14 (corresponding to 106 J) and 15 (124 J). Treatment was performed on the forehead, lateral zygoma, malar fat pad, dorsal arm, and back. The dispersive return electrode was placed on the back for each patient. On the forehead, the impedance readings (in ohms) averaged 282 at level 14 and 265 at level 15. On the zygoma, they averaged 236 at level 14 and 214 at level 15. On the malar fat pad, they averaged 228 at level 14 and 225 at level 15. On the dorsal arm, they averaged 324 at level 14 and 336 at level 15. On the back, they averaged 180 at level 14 and 172 at level 15 [25].

The authors noted that in a given cosmetic treatment zone, the measured impedance was similar at the two different energy levels examined, ranging from 3 to 22 ohms (mean 12.4 ohms) for all five zones. However, there was considerable inter-patient variation in the recorded impedances within a given cosmetic zone, with most variation in the arm zone. On the other hand, there was consistent ranking from the highest to the lowest impedance zones among all patients, with greatest impedance demonstrated on the dorsal arm, followed in decreasing order by the forehead, the medial and lateral cheeks, and the back. The authors pointed out that the impedance values recorded for a given treatment area were directly related to the distance of this area from the return electrode on the back. Thus the target area on the back has the lowest impedance, given its close proximity to the dispersion electrode that is also located on the back. In addition, the authors stressed that pre-treating a given area with a local anesthetic may change the physical properties of the treatment zone, thus affecting the energy delivered to it by the ThermaCool TC system, which does not alter the current in response to such tissue manipulation [25].

The use of topical anesthesia during non-ablative monopolar RF treatment was studied by Kushikata *et al.* in 2005. The investigators enrolled

84 female patients in the study, dividing them into three groups. Group A underwent RF treatment with topical anesthesia; group B was treated without topical anesthesia; group C had one side of the face treated with and one without topical anesthesia. Topical anesthesia was afforded by ELA-Max 5% lidocaine. Treatment was provided to the face, from the lower edge of the eyelid to the lower mandibular area, with a single non-overlapping pass using the ThermaCool TC device, with treatment settings determined based on the feedback on each individual patient's pain tolerance [32].

The authors found that the average highest and lowest treatment settings used in the group receiving topical anesthesia (Group A) were 14.3 and 12.21. Group B, which received no topical anesthesia, exhibited highest treatment settings averaging 14.2 and lowest averaging 12.04. Topical anesthesia thus produced no significant difference in treatment tolerance. Similarly, split-face application of topical anesthesia in Group C failed to significantly alter the subjects' pain threshold and allow for higher treatment fluences to be used. Furthermore, patient satisfaction surveys conducted at 3 months following treatment showed no significant difference between patients in groups A and B [32].

Objective improvement based on clinical and three-dimensional photography at 3 months following treatment showed that 25% of patients in group A, 21.4% of patients in group B, and 21.4% of patients in group C experienced a better than 75% improvement in facial skin laxity. The percentage of patients experiencing 50–74% improvement was 42.9% of patients in group A, 46.4% of patients in group B, and 42.9% of patients in group C. The percentage of patients experiencing 25–49% improvement was 21.4% of patients in group A, 25% of patients in group B, and 25% of patients in group C. Less than 24% improvement was experienced by 10.7% of patients in group A, 7.2% in group B, and 10.7% in group C. Side effects reported in the study included transient erythema and pruritus in two patients in group A, mild blistering in one patient in group B. These were not thought to be related to the use of topical anesthesia. The authors concluded that the use of topical anesthesia does not significantly impact on either patient satisfaction or on the ability to utilize higher fluences in the treatment of facial laxity. Rather, the efficacy of treatment is a function of the target tissue physical and morphologic characteristics [32].

In 2006, Weiss and colleagues performed a retrospective analysis of over 600 monopolar RF treatments (ThermaCool TC) performed in their practice between 2002 and 2006 for skin tightening. The first treatments in the period were conducted using the 1 cm^2 standard tip, 81–124 J/cm^2 fluences, and 1–3 passes. Subsequently, patients were treated with the 1 cm^2 "fast" tip, fluences of 62–109 J/cm^2, with initial pass performed over the entire treatment area, followed by 2–4 additional passes over areas of laxity concern. As the therapy algorithm further evolved, the investigators began treating patients using first the 1.5 cm^2 "big fast" tip and then the 3 cm^2 tip, with fluences of 75–130 J/cm^2 and two passes over the entire treatment area, with up to four additional passes performed over the areas of greatest laxity. The treatment fluence was adjusted so as to not exceed each individual patient's pain level of 2 on a scale of 0 (no pain or heat) to 4 (intolerable pain or heat) [19].

Side effects were reported to occur in 2.7% of patients treated by the device. These included erythema lasting 5–20 minutes in 90% of patients and up to 24–72 hours in 5%, edema lasting up to a day in 30% of patients and lasting up to 2 weeks in three patients, pain in the treated area lasting 2 days in 38% of patients, neck tenderness resolving in 1–4 weeks in three patients, subcutaneous erythematous acneiform papules in 3 patients resolving within 10 days, linear superficial crust formation in one patient resolving in 1 week, and a slight depression on the cheek resolving in 3.5 months in another patient. The authors reported that most significant side effects occurred with the use of the older 1 cm^2 treatment tip. No scarring, nerve injury, or pigmentary changes were reported. The authors reported a treatment efficacy of 20% using a single-pass technique with a slow 1 cm^2 treatment tip between 2002 and 2003; a 50% efficacy using a double pass treatment approach using the slow and fast 1 cm^2 tips between 2003 and 2004; and a 80% efficacy since 2004 with a multi-pass algorithm utilizing slow and fast 1 cm^2, "big fast" 1.5 cm^2, and the "bigger" 3 cm^2 tips [19].

In 2007, Dover et al. conducted a survey of 5700 patient monopolar RF facial skin tightening treatments by 14 physicians in four different specialties, including dermatologic surgery, plastic surgery, facial plastic surgery, and oculoplastic surgery, to determine whether patient feedback on heat sensation during therapy was a preferred method for optimal energy selection; whether a moderate-energy multiple-pass algorithm was efficacious, compared to the original high-energy single pass protocol; and whether treatment to a clinical endpoint of tightening was predictive of the clinical results [18].

The authors found that immediate tightening was reported in 87% of patients with the new lower-energy multi-pass algorithm, compared to 54% with the older higher-energy single-pass approach. The prevalence of skin tightening at 6-month follow-up was also higher with the new algorithm (92% vs. 54%). Compared to the older regimen, more patients reported treatment meeting their expectations using the new technique (94% vs. 68%), and fewer patients reported that the procedure was too painful (5% vs. 45%). The authors concluded that the use of the new lower-energy multi-pass algorithm, treating to an observed endpoint of tightening, provides a more effective treatment while minimizing patient discomfort [18].

In their 2007 study to evaluate the utility of the multiple-pass, low-fluence algorithm for monopolar radiofrequency treatment of lower facial laxity, Bogle and colleagues enrolled 66 male and female subjects, ages 40–75 (mean 53) with Fitzpatrick skin types of I–IV and moderate facial laxity of the AB (combined cutaneous and subcutaneous laxity) or B (subcutaneous laxity) type according to the Leal laxity classification system. Exclusion criteria included type A (solely cutaneous laxity) based on the "pinch test," non-existent (0), prominent (4), and extreme (5) laxity on a 0–5 scale [17].

The cheeks, perioral area, chin, submental region, and the upper neck were treated with five passes of non-stacked, non-overlapping pulses using the ThermaCool monopolar RF device using the 1.5 cm^2 tip, with delivered fluences not exceeding each patient's discomfort level of 2–3 on the 0–4 scale, averaging 83 J/cm^2. The number of pulses per treatment ranged from 220 to 720 (mean 480) [17].

Side effects reported in the study included mild transient erythema in two subjects, mild edema in one subject, mild transient superficial crusting in two subjects, focal linear depressions resolving within an hour in one subject, and jawline numbness resolving by 2 months in two subjects. No permanent complications were observed [17].

Patients were evaluated at 1, 2, 4, and 6 months following the treatment session on the basis of physical Leal laxity classification system, investigator assessment, independent photograph reviewers, patient evaluation, and the BTC2000 analysis, a biomechanical tissue characterization system measuring skin stiffness and energy absorption. The authors determined that at 4 months following treatment, 15% of patients experienced improvement the skin laxity defined in the Leal laxity system as moving from type B to type A or from type AB to either type A or type B laxity. This improvement increased further to 39% at 6 months. The authors determined that patients with type AB laxity at baseline were more likely than type B patients to experience improvement in the laxity type. The authors explained that this finding could be due to the greater degree of skin contraction afforded by both the dermal collagen and subcutaneous fibrous septae contraction in patients with combined AB laxity, compared to contraction in the subcuticular fibrous septae alone in patients with only deeper type B laxity [17].

At 4 months, the investigators noted improvement in the degree of laxity in 95% of patients, rating it very good (51–75%) in 19% and good (26–50%) in 46%. The percentage of patients showing skin laxity improvement at 6 months was 92%, with 28% showing very good and 33% showing good improvement. Interestingly, the group of patients treated with greatest number of treatment pulses (580) contained the largest number attaining very good improvement in laxity, compared to the group receiving the smallest number of treatment pulses (427), which had the fewest patients showing very good improvement and the most displaying minimal response, including the eight non-responders [17].

Independent photograph reviewers also noted improvement in the degree of laxity on the Leal scale in 75% of subjects at 4 months, and in 84% of subjects at 6 months. The most commonly improved facial region at 4 months was the lower face (48%), followed by the middle face (46%) and upper neck (32%). However, at 6 months, the reviewers found that the middle face most frequently showed improvement (65%), followed by the lower face (58%) and the upper neck (41%). The greater success of RF treatment seen in the middle and lower face may at least in part be explained by the relative abundance of subcutaneous adipose-containing treatment-responsive fibrous septae within the tissue of these regions, providing an added mechanism for skin tightening to dermal collagen contraction [17].

Patient satisfaction was reported at 78% 4 months following treatment, decreasing somewhat to 70% at 6 months. The BTC2000 analysis showed a significant increase in skin stiffness of 26 mmHg/mm at 2 months, the magnitude of which fell to 4 mmHg/mm at 4 months, and returned to baseline at 6 months. Energy absorption showed a decrease of 10.8 mmHg/mm at 2 months, followed by an increase of 0.2 mmHg/mm at 4 months and an increase of 3.6 mmHg/mm at 6 months. The analysis also showed that the percentage of patients experiencing an improvement in skin stiffness decreased steadily from 81% at 2 months to 71% at 4 months to 35% at 6 months. These findings were paralleled by the decrease in the number of patients showing improvement in skin energy absorption, from 81% at 2 months to 47% at 4 months to 25% at 6 months. The apparent lack of correlation between the physical data, showing a peak of improvement at 2 months followed by a decline in the subsequent follow-up periods, and the steadily increasing clinical improvement seen over time remains an unsolved conundrum pending further studies [17].

The authors also noted that, compared to earlier studies of Alster and Tanzi [33] and Nahm *et al.* [34], which utilized higher fluences and fewer pulses, the multiple-pass lower-fluence algorithm achieved superior improvement in the degree of skin laxity. The new treatment approach may also be associated with a lower risk of side effects and better patient tolerability [17].

The treatment of pronounced nasolabial folds has been approached by cosmetic surgeons in several ways, including dermal fillers to restore volume as well as through the use of non-ablative tissue-tightening devices to decrease facial laxity. Many clinicians utilize both approaches in order to provide a combination of an immediate response and long-term improvement. In 2007, Goldman and colleagues conducted a randomized trial to determine the clinical and histologic effects of a monopolar radiofrequency treatment (as well as treatment with non-ablative 1320 nm Nd:YAG and the 1450 nm diode lasers and intense pulsed light) performed immediately following administration of a hyaluronic acid gel agent. Of the 36 patients, ages 30–70 (mean 50), enrolled in the study, three received treatment using a monopolar RF ThermaCool TC device immediately following implantation of the Restylane® hyaluronic acid gel (Q-Medical AB, Uppsala, Sweden) in the ipsilateral nasolabial fold and postauricular region. The contralateral nasolabial fold and postauricular region received only the hyaluronic acid gel. Monopolar RF treatment was conducted using the 1.5 cm^2 treatment tip and 73–85 J/cm^2 energy density. The monopolar RF treatment was repeated using same parameters 2 weeks later [35].

The authors found no statistically significant difference in wrinkle severity scores or patients' global aesthetic improvement scores between the areas that received the combination hyaluronic acid and RF treatment compared to those that received hyaluronic acid alone. Histopathologic studies also showed no modification or disruption of the implanted hyaluronic acid by the monopolar RF treatment. Furthermore, no significant inflammation or additional side effects were elicited by combining the two treatment modalities. The authors conclude that the combination treatment with monopolar RF energy and hyaluronic acid dermal filler is a safe treatment option for management of pronounced nasolabial folds [35].

Likewise, skin laxity in the periocular areas is a major cosmetic concern presented to a cosmetic surgeon. Until recently, aesthetic blepharoplasty has been the sole method to combat this problem. Subsequently ablative and fractional laser resurfacing has added another method to the armamentarium. However, the significant recovery time after such procedures precludes many from undergoing these procedures. Non-ablative radiofrequency tightening has recently been studied for skin tightening of the eyelids and periocular areas [35].

In 2007, Jean and Alastair Carruthers performed a study to evaluate the efficacy and safety of the novel 0.25 cm^2 treatment tip of the ThermaCool TC monopolar radiofrequency device in the treatment of eyelid laxity. The study involved 20 patients with moderate eyelide skin laxity and hooding of the upper lids. Multiple passes were undertaken over the pretarsal, preseptal, and lateral orbital skin. Prior to treatment, a protective opaque black plastic haptic scleral contact lens (Oculo-Plastik Inc., Montreal, Quebec, Canada) was placed over the globe for ocular protection from the radiofrequency energy, following application of proparacaine HCl 0.5% ophthalmic anesthetic solution. Treatment was initiated at 12 J and increased based on the patient feedback, keeping the individual patient's comfort level below 2 on a 0–10 scale. Energies utilized ranged from 12 to14 J (32–34 treatment-level setting). Fifteen subjects underwent treatment to both upper and lower eyelids; one was treated on the lower eyelids and lateral orbital areas; four patients were treated on the upper eyelids and lateral orbital areas. Nineteen patients received five treatment passes, and one received eight passes [16].

At the 6-month follow-up visit, 87% of patients receiving upper eyelid treatment experienced at least a 25% tightening, with 3.33% of patient experiencing a 51–75% improvement. Lower eyelid tightening of at least 25% was seen in 67% of patients treated. The patient receiving eight treatment passes experienced the most significant tightening of the upper and lower eyelids. In contrast to evaluator assessment, subject satisfaction survey showed more patients satisfied with the lower eyelid treatment. One patient experienced punctuate epithelial erosions at the center of the corneal apex, which was attributed to the contact lens and resolved with topical antibiotic ointment within hours [16].

In an interesting 2007 study, Key performed a head-to-head split-face comparative analysis of a single treatment of monopolar RF and a long-pulsed 1064 nm Nd:YAG laser for treatment of facial laxity. Twelve female patients with Fitzpatrick skin types I and II were enrolled in this study. Both treatment sides were pre-treated with a topical anesthetic preparation composed of 20% benzocaine, 10% lidocaine, and 4% tetracaine. Patients received treatment with the ThermaCool TC monopolar RF device on one side of the face and with the GentleYAG long-pulsed 1064 nm Nd:YAG laser (Candela Corporation, Wayland, MA) treatment on the other side. The RF treatment was performed using fluences of 73–79 J/cm^2 (mean 75 J/cm^2), using the 1.0 cm^2 treatment tip, performing several passes without pulse stacking, for a total of 450 pulses. The laser treatment was performed using fluences of 20–30 J/cm^2 on the forehead and 40 J/cm^2 on the cheeks, with 50 ms pulse duration, 10 mm spot size, and 1.5 Hz 2-pulse stacking. Cooling was provided by Dynamic Cooling Device (Candela Corporation) set at 40/20/0 [36].

The patients were evaluated 2 months following treatment. Investigator assessment of clinical improvement in facial skin laxity on the upper face was 30.2% for the laser and 31.3% for the RF treatments, a difference that was not statistically significant. Lower face improvement of 35.7% on the laser-treated side was also insignificantly greater than the 23.8% on the RF-treated side. However, overall face improvement was found to be significantly greater on the laser-treated side (47.5%) compared with 29.8% on the RF-treated side. In addition, 58.3% of patients reported subjectively greater improvement on the laser-treated side, compared with the RF-treated side. Evaluators noted that 83.3% of patients had greater improvement on the laser-treated side of the face. All patients reported transient discomfort on the laser-treated side. No adverse effects were reported for either laser or RF-treated sides [36].

Alexiades-Armenakas and colleagues set out to compare the efficacy and safety of the unipolar and bipolar radiofrequency device for treatment of rhytides and skin laxity. In their 2008 study, 10 subjects aged 18–75 years underwent four treatment sessions 1 week apart, receiving therapy with unipolar and bipolar radiofrequency handpieces (Accent, Alma Lasers, Caesarea, Israel) in a split-face fashion. The bipolar RF handpiece provided 40.84 MHz of alternating RF current, eliciting volumetric heating to a depth of 2–4 mm into the reticular dermis, as a result of changing polarity orientation of the charged particles within the treated tissue. On the other hand, the unipolar handpiece effected tissue heating by generating a 40.84 MHz EMR, establishing an electromagnetic field up to 20 mm in depth, resulting in dipole water movement within the treated skin. Both treatments were carried out in 20-second passes, moving quickly across the treatment field with only gentle pressure application. The unipolar RF treatment, initiated at 90 watts, was continued for 1–2 passes until skin temperature peaked at 40 °C, then decreased by 10 watts for the first and again by 10 watts for the subsequent two maintenance passes. The bipolar RF treatment was initiated at 70 watts, followed by three 10-watt decremented maintenance passes. Contact cooling was also provided for epidermal protection [10].

Patients received follow-up at 1 and 3 months following treatment. The treatment with both devices was painless and well tolerated by the patients, with only minimal erythema resolving within 1–3 hours and no pigmentary changes, crusting, or scarring reported by the investigators. Although the authors found a tendency toward clinical improvement, they noted that this limited-pass protocol did not achieve statistical significance with either device. The unipolar device-treated side experienced a $6.0 \pm 4.6\%$ improvement in rhytides and $4.6 \pm 4.8\%$ improvement in laxity. On the bipolar device-treated side, a $4.4 \pm 2.5\%$ improvement in rhytides and $7.3 \pm 3.5\%$ improvement in laxity were noted. The authors noted that a 9–10 pass protocol may be superior in achieving a more favorable response, and that the mobile RF energy delivery method may be less likely than the stationary heat-delivery systems to be associated with pain and side effects, given the opportunity for cooling of the treated tissue below the 45 °C threshold at the dermoepidermal junction for firing of the A- and C-fiber nociceptors, while maintaing an adequate temperature for attaining collagen remodeling [10].

In their 2007 study, Friedman and Gilead evaluated the use of a hybrid radiofrequency device in the treatment of rhytides and lax skin. Sixteen female patients, ages 29–66 (mean 47) with Fitzpatrick skin types II–IV underwent 2–6 treatments (mean 4.3) with the Accent system at 2–3 week intervals. Eight patients received treatment to the forehead, seven in the periorbital area, twelve on the cheeks, six to the nasolabial folds, three to the marionette lines, five to the chin, and nine to the jowl lines. Twenty-three patients were treated for skin laxity and 27 were treated for rhytides. Unipolar RF treatments were performed during phase I at an average of

120 W × 20 s (1.6 kJ) per pass; and during phase II at 100 W × 20 s (2.4 kJ) per pass. Bipolar RF treatments were performed during phase I at an average of 60 W × 20 s (1.0 kJ) per pass; and during phase II at 50 W × 20 s (1.2 kJ) per pass. The unipolar treatment was conducted at a mean energy level of 120 ± 22 W and the bipolar at 60 ± 13 W. A 120-watt unipolar handpiece single-pass 20-second treatment over an area of 30 cm^2 resulted in an energy deposition of 80 J/cm^3. A single 20-second pass over an area of 30 cm^2 using a 60-watt bipolar handpiece deposited 40 J/cm^3 of energy. Temperature was monitored through the treatment using a laser thermometer (Center, 350 series, Center Technology Corp., Korea). The treatment was performed in two phases. During a non-therapeutic phase I, two treatment passes were undertaken to raise the baseline epidermal temperature to therapeutic level. Subsequently, in the therapeutic phase II, the target therapeutic temperature was maintained at 39–43 °C during three treatment passes. The authors noted that the baseline epidermal temperature of 31–33 °C increased to the therapeutic level of 42 °C in all areas within 2–3 passes [37].

One month following the last treatment, investigators noted significant (51–75%) improvement in rhytides and skin laxity in 42% of patients, and excellent (76–100%) improvement in 17% of patients. The authors noted that 44% of patients experienced significant and one patient excellent improvement in the appearance of the jowls. Significant improvement was also noted for forehead and periorbital rhytides in 37% of patients. Overall, 69% of patients experienced moderate to significant improvement and 19% showed marked (> 75%) improvement. A patient satisfaction survey conducted at 1 month following treatment showed that two patients reported excellent results, nine were satisfied to very satisfied, nine were somewhat satisfied to satisfied, and three were not satisfied or only somewhat satisfied with the improvement. The authors noted significantly better patient satisfaction in the younger patients treated by the device. The sole side effect reported in the study was transient post-treatment erythema resolving within 1–2 hours. No incidents of burns or scarring were reported [37].

In another recent study by Montesi and colleagues, the investigators evaluated the clinical efficacy and histopathologic and immunohistochemical changes associated with the treatment of facial rhytides, facial laxity with accentuation of the nasogenial furrow, and striae distensae using the Aluma bipolar RF device. Of the 30 patients, ages 18–70 (mean 44), enrolled in the study, four were treated for facial laxity. The treatment approach included treatment of the nasogenial furrow as well as at the preauricular region in order to affect vector-based superolateral movement of the cheek as a result of directed tissue tightening. The patients underwent 6–8 treatment sessions at 2-week intervals. Treatment parameters were 3-joule pulses (18 J total delivered energy), 3-second pulses with 3 seconds applied vacuum [26].

At the 3-month follow-up visit, two patients were noted to have 25–50% improvement in facial laxity and two showed less than 25% improvement. Transient erythema resolving within 12 hours was the sole reported adverse effect. Histological changes elicited by treatment using the bipolar RF system included increased dermal interstitital edema and decreased collagen atrophy. The authors noted that the degree of histologic improvement was dependent upon the age and the extent of the photodamage, with patients over the age of 60 with photoaged skin showing significantly less improvement than those with younger less photodamaged skin. Immunohistochemical examination using anticollagen I monoclonal antibodies showed a slight increase in collagen synthesis in the post-treatment biopsies. No changes in anticollagen III and anticollagen V monoclonal antibody staining was observed [26].

In a 2008 study by Carniol *et al.*, 10 female patients were treated with the Titan 1100–1800 nm infrared device. The patients underwent two treatments 1 month apart to the lower two-thirds of the face beginning at the inferior orbital rim to the upper two-thirds of the neck. Three passes at fluences of 34–36 J/cm^2 for the face and 33–34 J/cm^2 for the neck were undertaken, with patients reporting no pain, but only a warming sensation [27].

Compared with the baseline scores, the authors noted skin tightening at 1 month post-treatment that was further augmented by 3 months post-treatment, with greatest tightening occurring in the malar region (10% improvement from the baseline scores), the upper neck (10% improvement), and over the mandible (12% improvement). Patients participating in this study reported a 20% improvement in the appearance in the neck region, as well as a 32% improvement in the cheeks, and were satisfied with the treatment [27].

Another study of the infrared device in the treatment of facial skin laxity was conducted by Chan and colleagues in 2008. Thirteen Asian women underwent two treatments 4 weeks apart with the Titan infrared device to one side of the face, the other side serving as the control. Three passes were undertaken over the forehead, cheeks, and submental regions, using a 1.0 cm × 1.5 cm spot size. Treatment fluences were adjusted for each patient, so as to not exceed a moderate discomfort threshold, and ranged from 36 to 45 J/cm^2. Fluences were also reduced by 10–15% over the bony prominences, including the forehead [38].

The patients were evaluated subjectively using questionnaires and objectively via photograph assessment by two independent observers. Subjective patient evaluation showed that 23% of subjects had mild, 15% had moderate, and 54% significant improvement 3 months following treatment. Objective investigator evaluation showed 41% of patients with clinical improvement 3 months post-treatment. This improvement in skin laxity was found to be statistically significant. The only treatment-related side effect reported in the study was blistering occurring in one patient and resolving uneventfully 3 months following treatment. Among limitations of this infrared device system, the authors cited its relatively small spot size, compared to the $3 \text{ cm} \times 3 \text{ cm}$ spot size of the monopolar RF device, which along with a longer pulse duration (5–10 s) makes this device most suitable for more localized areas of laxity. They advocated a larger spot size infrared light device (Starlux, Palmonar, Burlington, MA) and the monopolar RF device for treating larger areas of the face and in the off-face locations [38].

Another study providing further support for the use of the non-ablative infrared light device in the treatment of facial and neck laxity was provided by Chua and colleagues in 2007. Twenty-one patients having Fitzpatrick IV and V Asian skin underwent a series of three treatments at monthly intervals using the Titan infrared device. Treatment was performed in three non-overlapping passes, over the cheeks and submental areas at $32\text{--}40 \text{ J/cm}^3$ and over forehead and bony prominences at $28\text{--}32 \text{ J/cm}^3$. The investigators reported that treatment resulted in minimal pain and edema [28].

At the 6-month follow-up visit, patient assessment of the improvement was mild in 19%, moderate in 38%, and good in 43%. Physician evaluation of clinical improvement in laxity was 28% mild, 28% moderate, and 19% excellent. Treatment-associated side effects reported in the study were superficial blistering in seven of 63 treatments, associated with transient post-inflammatory pigment alteration, which resolved uneventfully 6 months following treatment. The authors noted that these occurred when higher $36\text{--}40 \text{ J/cm}^3$ fluences were utilized. No side effects occurred when $28\text{--}34 \text{ J/cm}^3$ fluences were used [28].

In a study conducted by Ruiz-Esparza in 2006, involving 25 patients 44–75 years of age, with skin types I–V, the author evaluated the Titan infrared device for eyebrow lifting and lower face and neck tightening. Treatment was performed using $20\text{--}30 \text{ J/cm}^3$ fluences for 20 patients and 40 J/cm^3 for five patients, all at a $10 \text{ mm} \times 15 \text{ mm}$ spot size. Twenty patients underwent one treatment, four received two treatments, and one was treated three times [29].

All patients reported satisfaction with treatment. No pain was reported by patients at fluences below 30 J/cm^3. Eighteen of the 24 treated patients experienced eyebrow lifting; 18 of the 22 treated patients experienced improvement in the cheek and neck laxity. Improvement was characterized as excellent in 13 patients, moderate in three patients, and minimal in six patients. Three patients failed to show improvement in any treatment areas. The author reported that treatment utilizing $20\text{--}25 \text{ J/cm}^3$ fluences and less than 150 pulses did not yield significant clinical response, whereas therapy at 150–360 pulses at a fluence of 30 J/cm^3 produced moderate to excellent improvement. The investigator noted that of the 22 patients who experienced immediate tissue tightening following treatment, all retained this improvement both in the days following treatment and at 12 months after therapy. According to the author, this signifies that the immediate improvement following treatment with this infrared device derives primarily from collagen contraction, as opposed to the tissue edema that is comonly seen after treatment with non-ablative RF devices. Treatment-associated side effects reported in the study consisted of superficial second-degree burns in three of the treated patients, which healed without difficulty [29].

Further support for the use of the Titan infrared device came from Goldberg and colleagues in 2007, who conducted a study involving 13 female patients, ages 58–83 (mean 64), 12 of whom completed the study. Each patient received two treatments performed 1 month apart with the 1100–1800 nm Titan device, using fluences of 30–36 J/cm^2 based on patient tolerability, with most patients treated at 36 J/cm^2. The number of pulses ranged from 230 to 440 (mean 312). Three passes were performed over the treatment area. Contact cooling was provided using the sapphire tip and ultrasound gel before, during, and after each pulse, maintaining a surface temperature below 40 °C [13].

Patients were evaluated at 1, 3, and 6 months following the last therapy session. The investigators found significant improvement in the mandibular definition and decreased neck skin redundancy in patients having skin laxity which was distinct from the deeper underlying subcutaneous tissue, compared with mild to moderate improvement in those patients in whom subcutaneous tissue accompanied the skin envelope in its descent into the submandibular area. In the one patient who did not respond to treatment, the treated jowl region consisted primarily of subcutaneous fat with no excess skin. This study was the first of its kind to demonstrate that the infrared device technique may have significant impact on the treatment of laxity in older patients, a population group that has previously been considered relatively refractory to such treatment [13].

The ultrastructural effects of the Titan infrared device were recently evaluated by Zelickson and colleagues. In their 2006 study, cadaveric forehead skin was treated with the Titan device at fluences of 50 and 100 J/cm^2 using the 1 cm × 1.5 cm spot size, with 5–10 s pulse durations. Abdominal skin of a patient undergoing abdominoplasty was treated prior to surgery at fluences of 30, 45, and 65 J/cm^2, using the 1 cm × 1.5 cm spot size and 3–6 s pulse durations. Contact cooling was afforded by the sapphire contact cooling tip set at 20 °C [39].

Punch biopsies of the specimens were analyzed using transmission electron microscopy to evaluate changes on collagen fibrils. The authors evaluated collagen both for reversible changes, indicated by an increase in the collagen fibril diameter and boarder softening, and for irreversible change, signified by the loss of normal collagen fibril morphology associated with denaturation. In the forehead specimen, the greatest impact on collagen was seen in the 1–2 mm depth range using both fluences. In the abdominal specimen, collagen fibril changes were noted at both the 0–1 mm and 1–2 mm depth levels, with comparably more changes observed at higher fluences and greater depths. The depth of maximal damage, or centroid, occurred at the 1–2 mm level. These findings reflect the protection provided to the superficial skin layers by the cool sapphire tip [39].

In 2007, Yu *et al.* conducted a study involving 19 patients with Asian skin type III–V, in which they studied the clinical efficacy of the combined radiofrequency-infrared light device for the treatment of facial laxity and periorbital rhytides. The ReFirme ST Applicator provided broadband infrared light treatment using wavelengths of 700–2000 nm delivered at 10 W/cm^2 in conjunction with 70–120 J/cm^3 bipolar RF energies. Each patient received three treatment sessions 3 weeks apart [40].

At 3 months follow-up, investigator assessment of the clinical improvement was 26.3% in the periorbital areas, nasolabial folds, and upper neck, 47.3% in the cheek region, and 36.8% in the jowls. The subject assessment of the improvement was somewhat more favorable, with 89.5% improvement in laxity of the periorbital areas, cheeks, jowls, and upper neck, and 78.9% improvement in the nasolabial folds. Side effects reported in the study were mild pain in 78.9% and moderate pain in 15.8% of patients, especially in the periorbital areas and forehead, transient post-treatment erythema (100% of patients), edema (15.8%), and small superficial crusting of the forehead (7%). No scarring or post-inflammatory pigment alteration was noted by the authors [40].

A recent 2007 study conducted by Alexiades-Armenakas investigated the use of the 1310 nm diode laser (prototype; Candela Corporation, Wayland, MA) for non-ablative skin tightening. The laser provides variable depth of heating by allowing the operator control over the cooling temperature, afforded by the surface cold sapphire plate, as well as pulse duration. Twenty patients 40–65 years of age (mean 52.2) with Fitzpatrick skin types I–V were enrolled in the study and randomized into three groups. All three groups received three laser treatments at 2–4 week intervals. Group IA received three passes using an 18 mm spot size, 3 s pulse duration, 1 s pre- and post-pulse cooling to 2 °C, and fluence of 26 J/cm^2. Group IB received three identical-parameter 32 J/cm^2 passes using an 18 mm spot size, 5 s pulse duration, and 1 s pre- and post-pulse cooling to 2 °C. Group II was treated with three passes of varying parameters: the first pass was delivered using a 12 mm spot size, 1 s pulse duration, 1 s pre- and post-pulse cooling time, cooling temperature of 2 °C, and a fluence of 21 J/cm^2; the second pass was undertaken using an 18 mm spot size, 3 s pulse duration, 1 s pre- and post-pulse cooling time to 2 °C, and a 27 J/cm^2 fluence; the third pass was performed using 18 mm spot size, 1 s pulse duration, no pre- or post-cooling (25 °C), and a fluence of 8 J/cm [41].

Side effects reported in the study consisted of transient post-treatment erythema and edema. The mean pain level reported by the treated patients was 1.6 on a scale of 1–10. At 1-month follow-up, the investigators noted that 45% of patients experienced a decrease in skin laxity. At 3 months, the percentage of patients with decrease in cutaneous laxity increased to 53%. A mean improvement in laxity was 7.9% at 1 month and 11% at 3 months. Subject surveys showed that at 1 month 78% of patients reported at least a mild improvement in facial skin laxity and 68% of patients reported at least a mild improvement in the neck skin laxity. At 3 months, at least a mild improvement in the laxity was still reported by 63% of patients for the face and 61% for the neck [41].

Conclusion

As reflected by these studies, the field of non-ablative facial tightening has undergone many a significant change over the past years since its introduction into the field of cosmetic dermatology. The technology has been studied and continues to be studied extensively in order to achieve even greater levels of efficacy, and to ensure patient safety. The treatment algorithms are not set in stone, but rather remain dynamic as additional data emerge from the numerous studies conducted on the subject by devoted pioneers of these technologies. New devices are introduced and their efficacy ascertained and scrutinized in the setting of the existing systems. Undoubtedly, the field of non-ablative facial tightening will continue to expand and strengthen in order to fulfill the public demand for a less invasive, better tolerated, and a more "natural" cosmetic enhancement.

References

1 Dierickx CC. The role of deep heating for noninvasive skin rejuvenation. *Lasers Surg Med* 2006; **38**: 799–807.
2 Abraham MT, Vic Ross E. Current concepts in nonablative radiofrequency rejuvenation of the lower face and neck. *Facial Plast Surg* 2005; **21**: 65–73.
3 Sadick N, Sorhaindo L. The radiofrequency frontier: a review of radiofrequency and combined radiofrequency pulsed-light technology in aesthetic medicine. *Facial Plast Surg* 2005; **21**: 131–8.
4 Scidenfeld J, Kron A, Aronson N. Radiofrequency ablation of unresectable primary liver cancer. *J Am Coll Surg* 2002; **194**: 813–28.

5 Zuboy J. Radiofrequency ablation used to treat renal and adrenal tumors. *Curr Treat Opt Oncol* 2000; **1**: 93–4.

6 Trohman RG, Parrillo JE. Direct current cardioversion: indications, techniques and recent advances. *Crit Care Med* 2000; **28**: 170–3.

7 Baujat B, Krastinova-Lolov D, Blumen M, Baglin AC, Coquille F, Chabolle F. Radiofrequency in the treatment of craniofacial plexiform neurofibromatosis: a pilot study. *Plast Reconstr Surg* 2006; **1**: 1261–8.

8 Tasto JP, Ash SA. Current uses of radiofrequency in arthroscopic knee surgery. *Am J Knee Surg* 1999; **12**: 186–91.

9 Weiss RA, Weiss MA. Controlled radiofrequency endovenous occlusion using a unique radiofrequency catheter under duplex guidance to eliminate saphenous varicose vein reflux: a two year follow-up. *Dermatol Surg* 2002; **28**: 38–42.

10 Alexiades-Armenakas M, Dover JS, Arndt KA. Unipolar versus bipolar radiofrequency treatment of rhytides and laxity using a mobile painless delivery method. *Lasers Surg Med* 2008; **40**: 446–53.

11 Zelickson B, Kist D, Bernstein E, *et al.* Histological and ultrastructural evaluation of the effects of a radiofrequency based nonablative dermal remodeling device: a pilot study. *Arch Dermatol* 2004; **140**: 204–9.

12 Alster TS, Lupton JR. Nonablative cutaneous remodeling using radiofrequency devices. *Clin Dermatol* 2007; **25**: 487–91.

13 Goldberg DJ, Hussain M, Fazeli A, Berlin AL. Treatment of skin laxity of the lower face and neck in older individuals with a broad-spectrum infrared light device. *J Cosmet Laser Ther* 2007; **9**: 35–40.

14 Orringer JS, Voorhees JJ, Hamilton T, *et al.* Dermal matrix remodeling after nonablative laser therapy. *J Am Acad Dermatol* 2005; **53**: 775–82.

15 Sukal SA, Geronemus RG. Thermage: the nonablative radiofrequency for rejuvenation. *Clin Dermatol* 2008; **26**: 602–7.

16 Carruthers J, Carruthers A. Shrinking upper and lower eyelid skin with a novel radiofrequency tip. *Dermatol Surg* 2007; **33**: 802–9.

17 Bogle MA, Ubelhoer N, Weiss RA, Mayoral F, Kaminer MS. Evaluation of the multiple pass, low fluence algorithm for radiofrequency tightening of the lower face. *Lasers Surg Med* 2007; **39**: 210–17.

18 Dover JS, Zelickson B; 14-Physician Multispecialty Consensus Panel. Results of a survey of 5700 patient monopolar radiofrequency facial skin tightening treatments: assessment of a low-energy multiple-pass technique leading to a clinical end point algorithm. *Dermatol Surg* 2007; **33**: 900–7.

19 Weiss RA, Weiss MA, Munavalli G, Beasley KL. Monopolar radiofrequency facial tightening: a retrospective analysis of efficacy and safety in over 600 treatments. *J Drugs Dermatol* 2006; **5**: 707–12.

20 Fisher GH, Jacobson LG, Bernstein LJ, Kim KH, Geronemus RG. Nonablative radiofrequency treatment of facial laxity. *Dermatol Surg* 2005; **31**: 1237–41.

21 Kushikata N, Negishi K, Tezuka Y, Takeuchi K, Wakamatsu S. Non-ablative skin tightening with radiofrequency in Asian skin. *Lasers Surg Med* 2005; **36**: 92–7.

22 Abraham MT, Mashkevich G. Monopolar radiofrequency skin tightening. *Facial Plast Surg Clin North Am* 2007; **15**: 169–77.

23 Fitzpatrick R, Geronemus R, Goldberg D, Kaminer M, Kilmer S, Ruiz-Esparza J. Multicenter study of noninvasive radiofrequency for periorbital tissue tightening. *Lasers Surg Med* 2003; **33**: 232–42.

24 Ruiz-Esparza J, Gomez JB. The medical face lift: a noninvasive, nonsurgical approach to tissue tightening in facial skin using nonablative radiofrequency. *Dermatol Surg* 2003; **29**: 325–32.

25 Lack EB, Rachel JD, D'Andrea L, Corres J. Relationship of energy settings and impedance in different anatomic areas using a radiofrequency device. *Dermatol Surg* 2005; **31**: 1668–70.

26 Montesi G, Calvieri S, Balzani A, Gold MH. Bipolar radiofrequency in the treatment of dermatologic imperfections: clinicopathological and immunohistochemical aspects. *J Drugs Dermatol* 2007; **6**: 890–6.

27 Carniol PJ, Dzopa N, Fernandes N, Carniol ET, Renzi AS. Facial skin tightening with an 1100–1800 nm infrared device. *J Cosmet Laser Ther* 2008; **10**: 67–71.

28 Chua SH, Ang P, Khoo LS, Goh CL. Nonablative infrared skin tightening in type IV to V Asian skin: a prospective clinical study. *Dermatol Surg* 2007; **33**: 146–51.

29 Ruiz-Esparza J. Near painless, nonablative, immediate skin contraction induced by low-fluence irradiation with new infrared device: a report of 25 patients. *Dermatol Surg* 2006; **32**: 601–10.

30 Kulick M. Evaluation of a combined laser-radio frequency device (Polaris WR) for the nonablative treatment of facial wrinkles. *J Cosmet Laser Ther* 2005; **7**: 87–92.

31 Finzi E, Spangler A. Multipass vector (mpave) technique with nonablative radio-frequency to treat facial and neck laxity. *Dermatol Surg* 2005; **31**: 916–22.

32 Kushikata N, Negishi K, Tezuka Y, Takeuchi K, Wakamatsu S. Is topical anesthesia useful in noninvasive skin tightening using radiofrequency? *Dermatol Surg* 2005; **31**: 526–33.

33 Alster TS, Tanzi E. Improvement of neck and cheek laxity with a nonablative radio-frequency device: a lifting experience. *Dermatol Surg* 2004; **30**: 503–7.

34 Nahm WK, Su TT, Rotunda AM, Moy RL. Objective changes in brow postion, superior palpebral crease, peak angle of the eyebrow, and jowl surface area after volumentric radiofrequency treatment to half of the face. *Dermatol Surg* 2004; **30**: 922–8.

35 Goldman MP, Alster TS, Weiss R. A randomized trial to determine the influence of laser therapy, monopolar radiofrequency treatment, and intense pulsed light therapy administered immediately after hyaluronic acid gel implantation. *Dermatol Surg* 2007; **33**: 535–42.

36 Key DJ. Single-treatment skin tightening by radiofrequency and long-pulsed, 1064-nm Nd:YAG laser compared. *Lasers Surg Med* 2007; **39**: 169–75.

37 Friedman DJ, Gilead LT. The use of hybrid radiofrequency device for the treatment of rhytides and lax skin. *Dermatol Surg* 2007; **33**: 543–51.

38 Chan HH, Yu CS, Shek S, Yeung CK, Kono T, Wei WI. A prospective, split face, single-blinded study looking at the use of an infrared device with contact cooling in the treatment of skin laxity in Asians. *Lasers Surg Med* 2008; **40**: 146–52.

39 Zelickson B, Ross V, Kist D, Counters J, Davenport S, Spooner G. Ultrastructural effects of an infrared handpiece on forehead and abdominal skin. *Dermatol Surg* 2006; **32**: 897–901.

40 Yu CS, Yeung CK, Shek SY, Tse RK, Kono T, Chan HH. Combined infrared light and bipolar radiofrequency for skin tightening in Asians. *Lasers Surg Med* 2007; **39**: 471–5.

41 Alexiades-Armenakas M. Nonablative skin tightening with a variable depth heating 1310-nm wavelength laser in combination with surface cooling. *J Drugs Dermatol* 2007; **6**: 1096–103.

CHAPTER 5

Photodynamic Photorejuvenation

Michael H. Gold

Vanderbilt University Medical School, Nashville, TN, USA

Key points

- Photodynamic therapy (PDT), initially developed for the treatment of actinic keratoses, is now used to treat a variety of skin conditions
- PDT involves the use of a photosensitizer that is activated by a light source
- Although a limited number of photosensitizers are available, a wide array of light sources are currently used for PDT
- All patients treated with PDT are at risk for an associated photoreaction

---

Introduction

Photodynamic therapy (PDT) has become a mainstay in many dermatology offices treating a variety of cutaneous disorders including actinic keratoses and non-melanoma skin cancers, as well as the signs associated with photodamage.

Over the past decade, the rise of PDT in cutaneous medicine has been a welcome addition to the armamentarium of many physicians who treat patients with skin concerns. To witness its progress, from far-reaching thoughts and ideas, to implementation of the clinical trials which paved the way for PDT to become an established medical treatment, to the many new uses now being written about, has truly been a rewarding experience for those who have observed this therapy firsthand from the early days.

With new photosensitizers now available, and potentially with more to come, this therapy will continue to have a bright future in dermatology, dermatologic surgery, and throughout cutaneous medicine. This chapter will introduce the reader to PDT and its long and tortuous history, and describe our current understanding of its roles, as we continue to bring PDT to the forefront of our specialty. The photosensitizers used for PDT will also be described, and the peer-reviewed literature which supports their use will be reviewed. Finally, we will look at some of the potential photosensitizers which may play a role in the next generation of PDT.

Facial Resurfacing, 1st edition. Edited by David J. Goldberg. © 2010 Blackwell Publishing.

In order to understand PDT's role in photorejuvenation, we must also review PDT in the context of how it was first used in modern dermatology, in the treatment of actinic keratoses (AKs) and superficial basal cell carcinomas (BCCs). Through this discourse we will understand how PDT becomes useful as a treatment for photorejuvenation of the skin. As a basis to all of our understanding of PDT, we must know that for a successful PDT reaction to occur, three elements are required: a photosensitizer, an appropriate light source, and oxygen.

Historical background

PDT use can be traced to the beginning of the twentieth century, when Raab reported that paramecia cells (*Paramecium caudatum*) were unaffected after exposure to either acridine orange or light alone, but that they died within 2 hours of exposure to both the photosensitizer (acridine orange) and light given at the same time [1]. In 1904, Von Tappeiner and Jodblauer used the term "photodynamic effect" in describing an oxygen-consuming reaction process in protozoa after the application of aniline dyes with fluorescence [2]. The following year, Jesionek and Von Tappeiner used topical 5% eosin as a photosensitizer with an artificial light source to treat dermatologic entities in humans [3]. These included non-melanoma skin cancers, lupus vulgaris, and condylomata lata. It was postulated that the eosin was incorporated into the cells and produced a cytotoxic reaction when exposed to an appropriate light source and oxygen.

The use of porphyrins as photosensitizers for PDT soon became popular amongst researchers. In 1911, Hausman reported on the use of hematoporphyrin as a photosensitizer, demonstrating that light-activated hematoporphyrin could photosensitize both guinea pigs and mice [4]. In 1913, Meyer-Betz, attempting to demonstrate a PDT effect in humans, self-injected the hematoporphyrin and found that when the areas were exposed to light they became swollen and painful [5]. This phototoxic reaction lasted for two months, creating a problem for future investigators studying hematoporphyrin as a photosensitizer and attempting to use it in cutaneous medicine. For approximately the next 30 years the medical literature did not seem to have an interest in PDT, and slowly, after a short but exciting beginning, PDT seemed to disappear from medicine.

The next significant PDT contribution in the medical literature appeared in 1942, when Auler and Banzer showed that hematoporphyrin, used as a photosensitizer, would concentrate more in certain dermatologic tumors than in their surrounding tissues, and that when these tumors were fluoresced with a light source they would became necrotic [6]. Figge *et al.* later reported that hematoporphyrin was also selectively absorbed into other cells, including embryonic, traumatized skin, and neoplastic cells [7].

Table 5.1 Uses of photodynamic therapy in dermatology.

Actinic keratoses (AKs)
Photodamage and associated actinic keratoses*
Bowen's disease
Superficial basal cell carcinoma
Superficial squamous cell carcinoma
Cutaneous T-cell lymphoma
Kaposi's sarcoma
Malignant melanoma
Actinic chelitis
Keratoacanthoma
Psoriasis vulgaris
Human papillomavirus
Molluscum contagiosum
Alopecia areata
Hirsutism
Acne vulgaris*
Sebaceous gland hyperplasia*
Hidradenitis suppurativa*

* Common indications for 5-aminolevulinic acid (ALA) photodynamic therapy in the United States.

From these initial clinical contributions in the medical literature, the principles of PDT in human cancer cells was firmly established. A photosensitizer could be concentrated into tumor cells and activated by a light source, and in the presence of oxygen would cause a cytotoxic reaction to occur selectively in the tumor cells. In 1978, Dougherty *et al.* reported on a new photosensitizer, hematoporphyrin purified derivative (HPD) [8]. HPD was a complex mixture of porphyrin subunits and by-products. They showed that HPD, after exposure to a red light source, could be successfully used to treat non-melanoma skin cancers. Systemic HPD became the accepted photosensitizer for PDT at that time, and a variety of medical uses emerged for PDT over the next several years, both oncologic and non-oncologic (Table 5.1).

In 1990 Kennedy *et al.* introduced 20% 5-aminolevulinic acid (ALA), the first topically applied photosensitizer [9]. This was the major breakthrough for modern PDT, and has been the impetus for all of the clinical research which has followed. The ALA acted as a photosensitizer and is known as a prodrug. It had the ability to penetrate the stratum corneum and be absorbed by actinically damaged skin cells, by non-melanoma skin cancer cells, and by the pilosebaceous units of the skin. Kennedy *et al.* showed that once ALA is incorporated into a cell it is converted into its active compound, which allows the PDT reaction to occur.

ALA, once incorporated into the cells, is converted to protoporphyrin IX (PpIX). ALA, as shown in Figure 5.1, is the natural precursor of PpIX in the heme biosynthetic pathway. Figure 5.2 shows the absorption spectrum of

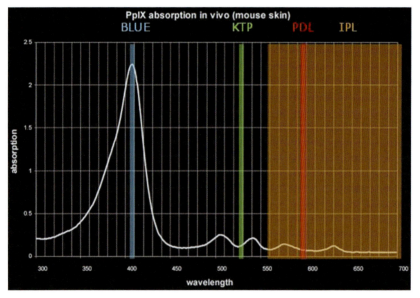

Succinyl-CoA

+

Glycine

δ – aminolevulinic acid synthase
(ALA synthase)

CO_2

Figure 5.1 Heme biosynthetic pathway.

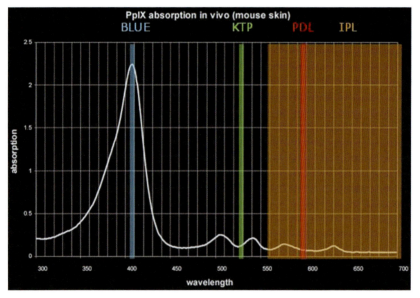

Figure 5.2 Protoporphyrin IX (PpIX) absorption spectrum. KTP, potassium titanyl phosphate; PDL, pulsed dye laser; IPL, intense pulsed light.

PpIX, with peak absorption bands identified in both the blue-light (known as the Soret band) and red-light spectra. Smaller peaks of energy are also seen throughout this absorption spectrum curve, and this is important, as much of the recent research on the use of PDT has centered on its ability to be utilized with a number of lasers and light sources, all falling within the absorption spectrum of PpIX, as demonstrated in Figure 5.2 [10].

The heme biosynthetic pathway (Fig. 5.2) is maintained under a close feedback loop, not allowing for buildup of heme or its precursors in tissues. Exogenous ALA has been found to be cleared from the body much more rapidly than HPD, so the potential for photoxicity from ALA-induced PpIX is greatly reduced, to only days, not months, as was the norm in years past. Thus ALA (or one of its derivatives) has become the main photosensitizer available for use in PDT today.

Recent developments

PDT in recent times has seen two distinct development pathways, which can be described as the American path and the European path. Throughout the 1990s and early in the 2000s there was a distinct separation, but it appears that the two paths are now converging, which will allow clinicians to determine which photosensitizer they want to use and will hopefully allow us to determine if, in fact, one may be better than the other for certain dermatologic entities.

In the American pathway, work has centered predominantly on 20% 5-ALA solution (Levulan® Kerastick®, DUSA Pharmaceuticals, Wilmington, MA). The primary indications for its use in the US market are to treat AKs with or without photorejuvenation, moderate to severe inflammatory acne vulgaris, sebaceous gland hyperplasia, and hidradenitis suppurativa. The Levulan Kerastick utilized is shown in Figure 5.3, and the blue light source used (BluU®, DUSA Pharmaceuticals) is shown in Figure 5.4.

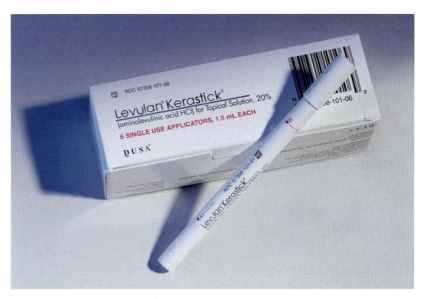

Figure 5.3 Levulan® Kerastick® (Dusa Pharmaceuticals, Wilmington, MA).

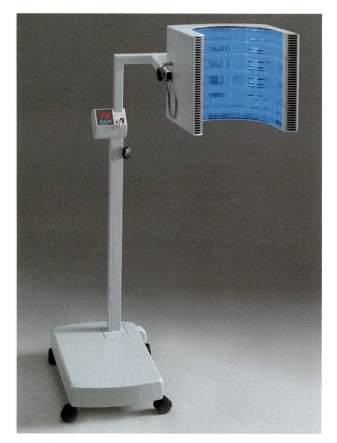

Figure 5.4 BluU® (Dusa Pharmaceuticals, Wilmington, MA).

The European pathway has centered on the methyl ester of 5-ALA (Metvix®, PhotoCure ASA, Norway; Metvixia®, Galderma, Ft. Worth, TX). Its primary use has been in treating non-melanoma skin cancers and AKs. Interest in photorejuvenation and inflammatory acne vulgaris has begun with methyl-ALA [10]. Metvix is shown in Figure 5.5 and the red light source currently available (Aktilite®, PhotoCure ASA, Norway; Metvixia, Galderma, Ft. Worth, TX) is shown in Figure 5.6.

Levulan, at the time of this writing, is available for use in the USA and has marketing rights assigned for Asia (Daewoong Pharmaceutical Co. Ltd, Seoul, South Korea) and South/Latin America (Stiefel Laboratories, Coral Gables, FL). The use of Levulan in Europe is currently being negotiated. Levulan has US FDA clearance for the treatment of non-hyperkeratotic AKs of the face and scalp utilizing a 14–18 hour drug incubation period of the ALA and using a blue light source for 16 minutes and 40 seconds (1000 seconds). All other indications being studied with Levulan are considered off-label use of the product.

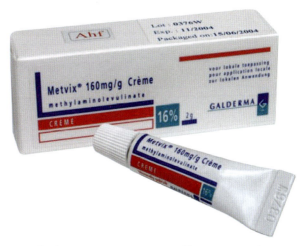

Figure 5.5 Metvix® (PhotoCure ASA, Norway; Galderma, Ft. Worth, TX).

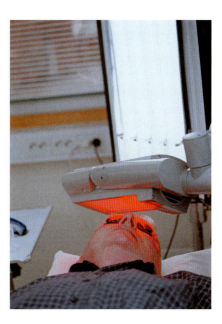

Figure 5.6 Red light source, Aktilite® (PhotoCure ASA, Norway; Galderma, Ft. Worth, TX).

Photorejuvenation: from the beginning

In order to understand the concept of photodynamic photorejuvenation, we also need to understand the concept of photorejuvenation in general, and what it means to those in dermatology and laser medicine.

Photorejuvenation refers to changes which are visible on the skin surface due to effects of years of sun/ultraviolet exposure and subsequent damage to skin cells. Nestor *et al.* reviewed the skin findings one typically sees in patients who present for the treatment of photodamage, a therapy described as photorejuvenation [11], and categorized photodamage as type I and type II.

Type I photodamage encompasses benign vascular lesions, including telangectasias, the symptoms of rosacea, and flushing of the skin. Type I photodamage also involves dyschromias or other pigmentary skin changes, erythema which follows laser resurfacing procedures, pigmentary sun damage, mottled hyperpigmentation, photoaging, and lentigines. These are all fairly superficial skin changes, easily handled with the proper therapy with the right medical device and proper skin care.

Type II photodamage brings in some of the deeper skin-care concerns that one sees associated with photodamaged skin. These include dermal and epidermal structural changes, rhytides, elastotic changes in the skin, collagenous and connective tissue changes, as well as the appearance of larger pores.

Conventional lasers and light sources, including intense pulsed light (IPL), can successfully combat the effects seen in both type I and type II photodamage. Much of the pioneering work into the use of IPLs stems from a study by Goldman and Eckhouse published in 1996, which described the first use of an IPL in the treatment of vascular lesions of the skin [12]. The IPL described then, and the premise of all IPL devices today, utilizes a broadband wave light to conform to the principle of selective photo-thermolysis, described several years earlier by Anderson and Parish [13]. That is, light can be selectively absorbed by a certain chromophore within the skin, destroy the target chromophore, and leave the surrounding tissues unaffected. The work by Goldman and Eckhouse [12] and others revolu-tionized the photorejuvenation market, and IPLs are now commonplace in many medical doctors' offices and medical spa settings.

IPLs are the mainstay in the photorejuvenation market of today. IPLs improve both the vascular problems of the skin and some of the pigmentary issues associated with photodamage. Furthermore, work done by Goldberg and Cutler [14] and Zelickson and Kist (personal communication) has shown that with an IPL device, changes in both the collagen and elastic tissue occur over time. Clinical trials over the years have demonstrated their effectiveness in skin types I–IV. Biter, in 2000, laid down the fabric for a photorejuvena-tion treatment when he reported that in the 49 individuals he studied, more than 90% of them had a greater than 75% improvement in rosacea symptoms (facial erythema and flushing), 84% had an improvement in their fine wrinkles, 78% had significant changes in their facial pigment, and 49% noted an improvement in their pore size [15]. Each one of the patients in this clinical trial received monthly full-face IPL treatments, up to five total treatments, similar to standards many of us continue to use to this day.

Other investigators also reported on their successes with photorejuvena-tion utilizing the IPL device. Goldberg and Samady evaluated 30 individuals and noted that one-third had substantial improvements with their series of IPL treatments, with one-half of the patients noting some improvement after the therapy [16]. Weiss *et al.*, in a retrospective analysis of IPL patients after 5 years, were able to demonstrate that improvement was maintained in skin texture (83%), telangectasias (82%), and skin dyschromias (79%) [17]. Sadick also examined changes in his patients treated with IPL, and found that more than 90% of individuals noted improvement in signs of photo-aging and in wrinkle appearance [18]. Other work by Negishi *et al.* has shown the effectiveness of the IPL in Asian skin types [19], and Hernandez-Perez has demonstrated similar results in Hispanic skin types [20].

Recent technological advances have improved the safety performances of the IPLs on the market. The IPL photorejuvenation procedures being performed today are safe and very predictable, yielding consistent results with little or no downtime for the patient. With IPL photorejuvenation well established, many investigators began to turn their attention to the possibilities offered by PDT.

Pivotal US trials for ALA-PDT: AKs

As indicated, the American path for PDT has been dominated over the years by ALA. The pivotal phase II US FDA clinical trial enrolled 39 patients with extensive non-hyperkeratotic AKs of the face and scalp. Each patient had the ALA individually placed onto their AKs and each patient received 16 minutes and 40 seconds of blue light after a 14–18 hour non-occluded drug incubation. Pain was noted by the majority of participants both dur-ing and after the treatment, and post-treatment erythema and edema, leading to crust formation for up to a week, was not uncommon. Eight weeks following treatment, however, 66% of the individually treated AKs resolved. A second treatment was given to the AKs that did not achieve a complete response, increasing the clearance rate to 85% during the follow-up period [21].

A phase III multicenter placebo-controlled clinical trial included 243 individuals with significant non-hyperkeratotic AKs on the face and scalp. Treatment parameters were the same as in the phase II trials, including individual AK treatment, a 14–18 hour drug incubation period, and 16 minutes and 40 seconds of blue-light therapy. Results from this study demonstrated > 70% complete clearance of individual AKs at 12 weeks. Again, for those AKs which had not cleared a second treatment was given, and at 24 weeks 88% of the individuals had ≥ 75% clearance of their AKs, compared to 20% in the placebo arm [22]. A clinical example from the phase III trial is shown in Figure 5.7. Pain was again noted by the majority of study participants, and downtime with healing was needed by most of

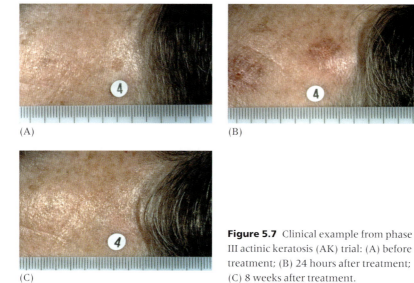

(A)

(B)

(C)

Figure 5.7 Clinical example from phase III actinic keratosis (AK) trial: (A) before treatment; (B) 24 hours after treatment; (C) 8 weeks after treatment.

the treated individuals. Downtime with healing has been termed the "PDT effect" by this author (MHG) and has been the subject of a great deal of interest in PDT research, as many of us have spent a great deal of our research time attempting to minimize this effect in our practices in the hope of making the therapy more palatable to many other clinicians. Of secondary significance during the phase III clinical trial was that 94% of the participants noted their cosmetic appearance as either good or excellent following their PDT treatment. Dermatologists interested in improving the cosmetic appearance of the skin began to take an interest in PDT and how it could be utilized more.

Open-label ALA-PDT clinical trials: AKs and photorejuvenation

In 2002, Gold reported early experiences with ALA-PDT utilizing a blue light source [23]. From the individuals studied, there appeared not only to be resolution of the treated AKs, but a positive response in contiguous areas to those being treated, resulting in a "rejuvenation" effect, as shown in Figure 5.8. A "PDT effect" was also quite evident in this series of patients, as they received ALA-PDT according to the original FDA label, including the long drug incubation and light exposure.

Alexiades-Armenakas and Geronemus reported in 2003 on the use of a long pulsed dye laser (PDL) in the treatment of AKs of the face and scalp [24]. They demonstrated the safety and efficacy of the PDL with ALA-PDT

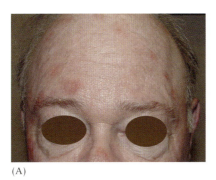
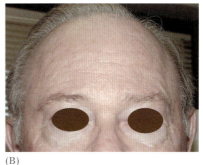

(A)   (B)

Figure 5.8 Rejuvenation effect after ALA-PDT: (A) before treatment; (B) after therapy; patient has received twice-yearly ALA-PDT for 7 years without the development of NMSC (non-melanoma skin cancer).

in the treatment of numerous AKs. They also were able to demonstrate that short-contact ALA (three hours) responded similarly to longer-contact drug incubation (14–18 hours) in the patients they were treating.

Shortly thereafter, several important papers appeared in the dermatologic literature which looked at (1) utilizing shorter ALA drug incubation times and (2) treating the entire face with ALA, potentially affecting both clinical and subclinical AKs and giving a full rejuvenation effect. Touma *et al.* clearly demonstrated that a 1-hour drug incubation time was as efficacious as the traditional incubation period of 14–18 hours in improving AKs and the parameters of photodamage with a blue light source [25]. Eighteen patients were evaluated in this clinical study, and improvements were seen in the sallowness of the skin, fine wrinkling, and mottled hyperpigmentation with a 1-hour drug incubation.

The second crucial clinical trial was reported by Ruiz-Rodriguez *et al.*, who also evaluated a shorter drug incubation time (3 hours) but used an IPL as a light source, the recognized leader in photorejuvenation lasers and light sources [26]. They treated 17 patients with an IPL device (full face treatments) and showed that after two ALA-IPL sessions the cosmetic appearance of the skin was excellent. All of the AKs cleared with the IPL-PDT therapy, and they showed an 87% improvement in skin texture, wrinkling, pigmentary changes, and telangectasias. Several other open-label clinical trials also have appeared in the dermatology literature that reinforced those trials already noted.

Gold *et al.* utilized a short drug incubation time of 30–60 minutes in 10 patients who had their full faces treated with ALA and a high-intensity blue light source [27]. They found that 83% of all AKs responded to the therapy. In addition, there was improvement in crow's feet in 90%, in skin roughness in 100%, in hyperpigmentation in 90%, and in facial erythema in 70%. Goldman *et al.* looked at blue light and a 1-hour drug incubation in

32 patients with AKs and photodamage [28]. They noted that 90% of the AKs responded to this therapy, and found improvement in skin texture in 72% and pigment changes in 59%. In addition, they found that 62.5% of their patients who had had previous cryotherapy for their AKs preferred PDT over cryotherapy. Avram *et al.* looked at an IPL device in 17 patients with a 1-hour full-face drug incubation [29]. In this study, 69% of the AKs responded with one IPL treatment, as well as an improvement of 55% in telangectasias, 48% in pigmentary changes, and 25% in skin texture. Alexiades-Armenakas and Geronemus studied 19 individuals with actinic cheilitis, using a PDL, and showed a 68% clearance at 12 months in these individuals [30]. All of these studies supported the use of ALA-PDT in treating AKs, actinic cheilitis, and the signs of photodamage, all with fewer treatments than with other modalities, and demonstrated the effectiveness of short-contact, full-face therapy with ALA-PDT.

Split-face clinical trials in the USA: AKs and photorejuvenation

Having open-label clinical trials is important in helping to define a concept and in bringing a therapy on its way to acceptance, but more rigorous clinical trials are necessary for the hypothesis to be proven. In the case of ALA-PDT, this required split-face clinical trials with the various lasers and light sources that appeared to be successful in PDT. All of the clinical trials reviewed below utilized short-contact, full-face therapy for their ALA-PDT treatments.

Five split-face US clinical trials have been published in the peer-reviewed medical literature. The first, by Alster *et al.*, compared ALA-IPL on one side of the face with IPL alone on the other side of the face in 10 individuals [31]. The group found that the combination of ALA and IPL improved the parameters of photorejuvenation compared to the side treated with IPL alone. Key examined subjects utilizing a PDL with ALA on one half of the face abd PDL alone on the other [32]. The ALA-PDL side showed improved parameters of photorejuvenation compared with the PDL side. Marmur *et al.* studied ALA-IPL versus IPL alone, and through skin biopsies examined ultrastructural changes, specifically looking at the production of type I collagen [33]. They found that there was a greater increase in type I collagen production with ALA-IPL than with IPL alone.

Dover *et al.* followed an ALA-IPL split face protocol in which patients received three split-face ALA-IPL treatments at 3-week intervals followed by two additional IPL full-face treatments, and then evaluated the patients 4 weeks after their last IPL treatment [34]. Twenty individuals participated in this clinical trial, and pre-treatment with ALA resulted in more improvement in the global score for photoaging (80% vs. 45%), mottled hyperpigmentation

(95% vs. 60%), and improvement in fine lines (60% vs. 25%) than IPL treatment alone. The authors found no statistical difference between ALA-IPL and IPL alone in tactile skin roughness or sallowness.

Gold *et al.* reported a split-face clinical trial utilizing ALA-IPL on one half of the face and IPL alone on the other half in 13 individuals [35]. Three split-face treatments at 4-week intervals, with follow-up at 1 and 3 months after the last treatment, were performed. They found changes in the ALA-IPL side versus the IPL side consisting of improvements in AKs (78% vs. 53.6%), crow's feet (55% vs. 28.5%), tactile skin roughness (55% vs. 29.5%), mottled hyperpigmentation (60.3% vs. 37.2%), and in improvement in erythema (84.6% vs. 53.8%). No adverse effects were noted and no "PDT effect" was seen.

All of these clinical trials confirmed the use of a short-contact, full-face ALA-PDT in the treatment of AKs and in photorejuvenation, thus completing the American path for the development of ALA-PDT as a therapy for AKs and for photorejuvenation. Many clinicians are utilizing this therapy on a regular basis in their clinical practices, and many patients have responded positively. Although there are no conclusive clinical studies to determine the optimal drug incubation for ALA-PDT, most clinicians utilize a 1-hour incubation time for ALA to be on the skin before exposure to a laser or light source. Clinical examples of responses to ALA-PDT are shown in Figures 5.9 and 5.10.

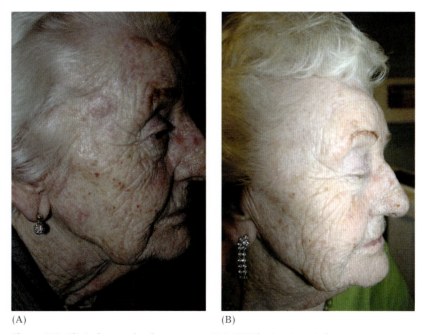

(A)   (B)

Figure 5.9 Clinical example of response to ALA-PDT for treatment of AKs/photorejuvenation: (A) before treatment; (B) after two ALA-PDT treatments.

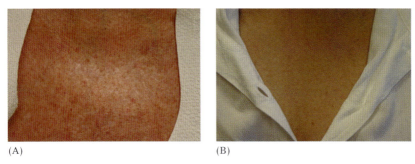

(A)   (B)

Figure 5.10 Clinical example of response to ALA-PDT for AKs/photorejuvenation:
(A) before treatment; (B) after three ALA-PDT treatments.

Two other important clinical papers have recently been published. The first, by Tschen *et al.*, looked at recurrence rates for AKs following ALA-PDT and found that with the therapy, new AK lesion development was significantly delayed [36]. In the second, Redbord and Hanke looked at complication rates following ALA-PDT therapy in a clinical practice setting, and found only two complications in over 200 PDT treatments, in each case a phototoxic reaction [37].

Metvix/Metvixia: the methyl ester of ALA for AKs, non-melanoma skin cancers, and photorejuvenation

The European pathway for PDT has focused its energy on a second photo-sensitizer, known as Metvix/Metvixia. Metvix/Metvixia, or MAL, is the methyl ester of ALA and is currently being used in PDT therapy throughout Europe and Australia. It has European Union (EU) clearance for the treatment of non-hyperkeratotic AKs of the face and scalp and BCCs that are not suitable for conventional surgery. Numerous clinical trials have been published to demonstrate the efficacy of this product in the treatment of AKs, Bowen's disease, and non-melanoma skin cancers, with skin cancer data showing efficacy results at 5 years. These are summarized in Table 5.2.

In the USA, two important phase III clinical trials have demonstrated the safety and efficacy of MAL in the treatment of AKs [45,46]. Both of these clinical trials utilized a similar clinical protocol, which involved lesion preparation of the AKs by gentle curettage, 3 hours of drug incubation under occlusion, and exposure to a red light source at 630 nm and a light dose of 37 J/cm^2 (Fig. 5.11) for 8 minutes. Therapy consisted of two treatments at 1-week intervals with follow-up at 3 months after the last treatment. MAL was found to be superior to vehicle with respect to complete lesion response (86.2% vs. 52.2%) and patient complete response (59.2% vs. 14.9%) in the first US trial [45]. MAL is now FDA-approved for

Table 5.2 Summary of clinical experience of Metvix for AKs.

Study	No. of patients (no. treated with Metvix)	No. of lesions treated with MAL PDT	Dosage regimen	Results (lesion complete response, CR) at 3 months
Phase II study (Braathen) [38]	110 (110)	384	Dose and regime finding study	Metvix 160 mg/g for 3 hours optimal (compared: 1 and 3 hours, 80 and 160 mg/g)
				Second Metvix PDT increased CR from 67% to 89% (lesions were prepared)
				Efficacy is better with lesion preparation than without
1 × Metvix PDT vs. double freeze–thaw cryotherapy (Szeimies) [39]	202 (102)	367	1 × MAL PDT session	Complete lesion response at 3 months: 1 × Metvix session (69%) as effective as double freeze–thaw cryotherapy (75%)
			For lesions on face & scalp (93% of lesions)	96% of patients had excellent or good cosmetic outcome vs. 81% with cryotherapy
			vs. double cycle cryotherapy	74% of patients preferred Metvix PDT to previous other therapies
European double-blind, placebo-controlled trial (Bjerring) [40]	39 (39)		1 × MAL PDT session	Complete lesion response at 3 months: 1 × Metvix session (76%) > placebo (18%)
			vs. placebo	
2 × Metvix PDT vs. single cryotherapy, placebo-controlled (Freeman) [41]	200 (88)	295	2 × MAL PDT sessions 7 days apart	Complete lesion response at 3 months: 2 × Metvix sessions (91%) > cryotherapy (68%) > placebo (30%)
			vs. single cycle cryotherapy	84% of patients had an excellent cosmetic outcome with Metvix PDT vs. cryotherapy (51%)
				98% had excellent or good cosmesis with Metvix
				85% of patients rated Metvix better (61%) or equal (14%) to previous treatments

Table 5.2 (*continued*)

Study	No. of patients (no. treated with Metvix)	No. of lesions treated with MAL PDT	Dosage regimen	Results (lesion complete response, CR) at 3 months
US double-blind, 2 × Metvix PDT vs. placebo-controlled trial (Pariser) [42]	80 (42)	260	2 × MAL PDT sessions 7 days apart vs. placebo	Complete lesion response at 3 months: 2 × Metvix sessions (89%) > placebo (38%) 97% of patients had excellent or good cosmetic outcome with Metvix PDT 73% of patients preferred Metvix PDT to other previous therapies
Single Metvix PDT vs. dual Metvix PDT (Tarstedt) [43]	211 (105)	400	1 × MAL PDT session, re-treat only non-complete responding lesions at 3 months (19%) (regime I) vs. 2 × MAL PDT 7 days apart (regime II)	At 3 months : for thin lesions, complete lesion response similar with 1 × Metvix (93%) and 2 × Metvix (89%); for thicker lesions, CR better with 2 × Metvix (84%) > 1 × Metvix (70%), which improved after repeat treatment at 3 months (88%) Regime I not inferior to regime II Overall: regime I: 92% (81% after first session); regime II: 87% For thin lesions: regime I 97%; regime II 89% For thicker lesions: regime I: 88%; regime II: 84%
Intra-individual (right–left) comparison 1 × Metvix PDT vs. double cryotherapy (Aktion Study, Morton) [44]	119 (119)	758	1 × MAL PDT session vs. double freeze–thaw cryotherapy, Non-complete responding lesions re-treated at 3 months MAL PDT 14.9% Cryotherapy 26.8%	Complete lesion response at 3 months:1 × Metvix session 83%; double freeze–thaw cryotherapy 72% Half as many lesions (10% vs. 20%) required re-treatment at 3 months with Metvix to achieve similar CR rates at 6 months (86% Metvix PDT vs. 83% cryotherapy) "Excellent" cosmetic outcome: Metvix PDT 71%; cryotherapy 57% Overall patient preference was significantly higher with Metvix (45% vs. 10%; $p < 0.001$)

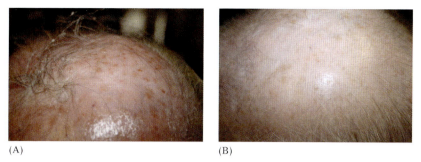

(A)   (B)

Figure 5.11 MAL-PDT clinical example: (A) before treatment; (B) after two treatments with Metvix and Aktilite.

the treatment of non-hyperkeratotic AKs of the face and scalp, and has just become available in the US market. MAL is not FDA-approved in for the treatment of BCCs.

A PDT effect is usually reported with most of these treatments, most likely as a result of the longer drug incubation period currently being utilized, and because of the deeper penetrating red light source. Comparative clinical trials utilizing Levulan in a 1-hour drug incubation, as is the standard used in the USA today, and with Metvix, utilizing the 3-hour drug incubation, have not been performed to determine differences between efficacy and adverse events. There also have been three reported cases of allergic contact dermatitis to MAL [47–49], and this remains a worry for those utilizing this therapy. In the first report, patch testing showed an allergic response to the MAL but not the ALA. An intense contact dermatitis reaction was noted in all of the examples of allergy.

Clinical trials for photorejuvenation with MAL have begun. Many investigations are being performed by colleagues from around Europe, looking at AKs and photorejuvenation. The first, by Seit in 2006, evaluated a group of patients who received a 1-hour drug incubation of MAL followed by treatment with red light [50]. He found that there was an 86% resolution of AKs, 50% improvement in telangectasias, 57% improvement in pigmentary changes, 52% improvement in skin texture, and a 33% improvement in skin tightening. This was with one MAL-PDT therapy.

Zane *et al.* looked at 20 patients with 137 AKs and severe photodamage [51]. In their protocol, patients received 3 hours of drug incubation under occlusion followed by red-light therapy. Two treatments were given to each patient. They found an 83.3% clearance of the AKs after two treatments, as well as improvement in photoaging, mottled hyperpigmentation, fine lines, roughness, and the sallowness of the skin. Most agree that in order for MAL to be successful in the cosmetic arena, variations in the parameters will have to be performed to minimize the PDT effect as far as possible.

Ruiz-Rodriguez *et al.* in 2006 reported preliminary findings with MAL for photorejuvenation utilizing a red light [52]. Ruiz-Rodríguez *et al.* in 2008 presented the formal results of this clinical trial [53]. It was a split-face, randomized clinical trial in which 10 patients received either 1 hour or 3 hours MAL drug incubation before therapy with red light. Three total treatments were given to each patient, and follow-up was for 2 months following the last treatment. The authors found a moderate improvement in fine lines, tactile roughness, and skin tightness in most of the patients, with more pronounced effects occurring in those receiving the 3-hour drug incubation. They found no changes in telangectasias or mottled hyperpigmentation. Adverse effects, especially erythema, edema, and scaling, were more pronounced on the 3-hour drug incubation group. AKs were successfully treated in all of the patients.

In a recent clinical trial, Goldman (personal communication) has performed a clinical trial in which patients were randomized to receive either blue light or red light following a 1-hour drug incubation with MAL. In this clinical trial, no significant differences were noted in the parameters of photorejuvenation utilizing the different light sources.

Thus we have now completed the European pathway for PDT, on its way to be molded into an American path. MAL-PDT is being utilized by US clinicians for the treatment of AKs and photodamage, as we have done with ALA-PDT.

Conclusion

Both ALA-PDT and MAL-PDT are becoming more widespread in the treatment of AKs and the signs of photodamage. Clinical trials have borne out their effectiveness, and patients are benefiting from this therapy on a daily basis. Further clinical uses still need to be defined, including a potential chemopreventive effect for PDT in immunosuppresed patients susceptible to numerous AKs and non-melanoma skin cancers. Research in this arena is now under way and may be very useful as PDT continues its growth in the USA.

References

1 Raab O. Ueber die wirkung fluoreszierenden stoffe auf infusorien. *Z Biol* 1900; **39**: 524–6.
2 Von Tappeiner H, Jodblauer A. Uber die wirkung der photodynamischen (fluorescierenden) staffe auf protozoan und enzyme. *Dtsch Arch Klin Med* 1904; **80**: 427–87.
3 Jesionek A, Von Tappeiner H. Behandlung der hautcarcinome nut fluorescierenden stoffen. *Dtsch Arch Klin Med* 1905; **85**: 223–7.

4   Hausman W. Die sensibilisierende wirkung des hamatoporphyrins. *Biochem Zeit* 1911; 276–316.

5   Meyer-Betz F. Untersuchungen uber die bioloische (photodynamische) wirkung des hamatoporphyrins und anderer derivative des blut-und gallenfarbstoffs. *Dtsch Arch Klin Med* 1913; **112**: 476–503.

6   Auler H, Banzer G. Untersuchungen ueber die rolle der porphyrine bei geschwulstkranken menschen und tieren. *Z Krebsforsch* 1942; **53**: 65–8.

7   Figge FHJ, Weiland GS, Manganiello LDJ. Cancer detection and therapy. Affinity of neoplastic embryonic and traumatized tissue for porphyrins and metalloporphyrins. *Proc Soc Exp Biol Med* 1948; **68**: 640.

8   Dougherty TJ, Kaufman JE, Goldfarb A, Weishaupt KR, Boyle D, Mittleman A. Photoradiation therapy for the treatment of malignant tumors. *Cancer Res* 1978; **38**: 2628–35.

9   Kennedy JC, Pottier RH, Pross DC. Photodynamic therapy with endogenous protoporphyrin IX: basic principles and present clinical experiences. *J Photochem Photobiol B* 1990; **6**: 143–8.

10 Gold MH, Goldman MP. 5-Aminolevulinic acid photodynamic therapy: where we have been and where we are going. *Dermatol Surg* 2004; **30**: 1077–84.

11 Nestor MS, Goldberg DJ, Goldman MP, Weiss RA, Rigel DS. Photorejuvenation: nonablative skin rejuvenation using intense pulsed light. *Skin Aging* 2003; **3**: 8.

12 Goldman M, Eckhouse S. Photothermal sclerosis of leg veins. *Dermatol Surg* 1996; **22**: 323–30.

13 Anderson RR, Parish JA. Selective photothermolysis: precise microsurgery by selective absorption of pulsed radiation. Science 1983; **220**: 524–7.

14 Goldberg DJ, Cutler KB. Non-ablative treatment of rhytids with intense pulsed light. *Lasers Surg Med* 2000; **26**: 196–200.

15 Biter PH. Noninvasive rejuvenation of photodamaged skin using serial, full-face intense pulsed light treatments. *Dermatol Surg* 2000; **26**: 835–42.

16 Goldberg DJ, Samady JA. Intense pulsed light and Nd:YAG laser non-ablative treatment of facial rhytids. *Lasers Surg Med* 2001; **28**: 141–4.

17 Weiss RA, Weiss MA, Beasley KL. Rejuvenation of photoaged skin: 5 years results with intense pulsed light of the face, neck and chest. *Dermatol Surg* 2002; **28**: 115–19.

18 Sadick NS. Update on non-ablative light therapy for rejuvenation: a review. *Lasers Surg Med* 2003; **32**: 120–8.

19 Negishi K, Tezuka Y, Kushikata N, Wakamatsu S. Photorejuvenation for Asian skin by intense pulsed light. *Dermatol Surg* 2001; **27**: 627–31.

20 Hernandez-Perez E. Gross and microscopic findings in patients submitted to nonablative full-face resurfacing using intense pulsed light: a preliminary study. *Dermatol Surg* 2002; **28**: 651–5.

21 Jeffes EW, McCullough JL, Weinstein GD, *et al.* Photodynamic therapy of actinic keratoses with topical aminolevulinic acid hydrochloride and fluorescent blue light. *J Am Acad Dermatol* 2001; **45**: 96–104.

22 Piacquadio DJ, Chen DM, Farber HF, *et al.* Photodynamic therapy with aminolveulinic acid topical solution and visible blue light in the treatment of multiple actinic keratoses of the face and scalp. *Arch Dermatol* 2004; **140**: 41–6.

23 Gold MH. The evolving role of aminolevulinic acid hydrochloride with photodynamic therapy in photoaging. *Cutis* 2002; **69** (6 Suppl): 8–13.

24 Alexiades-Armenakas MR, Geronemus RG. Laser-mediated photodynamic therapy of actinic keratoses. *Arch Dermatol* 2003; **139**: 1313–20.

25 Touma D, Yaar M, Whitehead S, Konnikov N, Gilchrest BA. A trial of short incubation, broad-area photodynamic therapy for facial actinic keratoses and diffuse photodamage. *Arch Dermatol* 2004; **140**: 33–40.

26 Ruiz-Rodriguez R, Sanz-Sanchez T, Cordoba S. Photodynamic photorejuvenation. *Dermatol Surg* 2002; **28**: 742–4.

27 Gold MH, Bridges TM, Bradshaw VL, Boring M. ALA/PDT and blue light therapy for hidradenitis suppurativa. *J Drugs Dermatol* 2004; **3**: S32–5.

28 Goldman MP, Atkin D, Kincad S. PDT/ALA in the treatment of actinic damage: real world experience. *Lasers Surg Med* 2002; **14** (Suppl): 24.

29 Avram DK, Goldman MP. Effectiveness and safety of ALA-IPL in treating actinic keratoses and photodamage. *J Drugs Dermatol* 2004; **3**: S36–9.

30 Alexiades-Armenakas MR, Geronemus RG. Laser-mediated photodynamic therapy of actinic cheilitis. *J Drugs Dermatol* 2004; **3**: 548–51.

31 Alster TS, Tanzi EL, Welsh EC. Photorejuvenation of facial skin with topical 20% 5-aminolevulinic acid and intense pulsed light treatment: a split-face comparison study. *J Drugs Dermatol* 2005; **4**: 35–8.

32 Key DJ. Aminolevulinic acid-pulsed dye laser photodynamic therapy for the treatment of photoaging. *Cosmet Derm* 2005; **18**: 31–6.

33 Marmur ES, Phelps R, Goldberg DJ. Ultrastructural changes seen after ALA-IPL photorejuvenation: a pilot study. *J Cosmet Laser Ther* 2005; **7**: 21–4.

34 Dover JS, Bhatia AC, Stewart B, Arndt KA. Topical 5-aminolevulinic acid combined with intense pulsed light in the treatment of photoaging. *Arch Dermatol* 2005; **141**: 1247–52.

35 Gold MH, Bradshaw VL, Boring MM, Bridges TM, Biron JA. Split-face comparison of photodynamic therapy with 5-aminolevulinic acid and intense pulsed light versus intense pulsed light alone for photodamage. *Dermatol Surg* 2006; **32**: 795–801.

36 Tschen EH, Wong DS, Pariser DM, *et al.* Photodynamic therapy using aminolaevulinic acid for patients with nonhyperkeratotic actinic keratoses of the face and scalp: phase IV multicentre clinical trial with 12-month follow up. *Br J Dermatol* 2006; **155**: 1262–9.

37 Redbord KP, Hanke CW. Topical photodynamic therapy for dermatologic disorders: results and complications. *J Drugs Dermatol* 2007; **6**: 1197–202.

38 Braathen L, Paredes B, Frolich K, *et al.* A dose finding study of photodynamic therapy (PDT) with Metvix in actinic keratosis (AK). *J Eur Acad Dermatol* 2000; **14**: 38.

39 Szeimies RM, Karrer S, Radakovic-Fijan S, *et al.* Photodynamic therapy using topical methyl 5-aminolevulinate compared with cryotherapy for actinic keratosis: a prospective, randomized study. *J Am Acad Dermatol* 2002; **47**: 258–62.

40 Bjerring P, Funk J, Poed-Petersen J, *et al.* Randomized double blind study comparing photodynamic therapy (PDT) with Metvix® to PDT with placebo cream in actinic keratosis. Abstract, 29th Nordic Congress of Dermatology and Venereology, Gothenburg, June 2001.

41 Freeman M, Vinciullo C, Francis D, *et al.* A comparison of photodynamic therapy using topical methyl aminolevulinate (Metvix®) with single cycle cryotherapy in patients with actinic keratosis: a prospective, randomized study. *J Dermatolog Treat* 2003; **14**: 99–106.

42 Pariser DM, Lowe NJ, Stewart DM, *et al.* Photodynamic therapy with topical methyl aminolevulinate (Metvix®) is effective and safe in the treatment of actinic keratosis: results of a prospective randomized trial. *J Am Acad Dermatol* 2003; **48**: 227–32.

43 Tarstedt M, Rosdahl I, Berne B, Svanberg K, Wennberg AM. A randomized multicenter study to compare two treatment regimens of topical methyl aminolevulinate (Metvix)-PDT in actinic keratosis of the face and scalp. *Acta Derm Venereol* 2005; **85**: 424–8.

44 Morton C, Horn M, Leman J, *et al.* Comparison of topical methyl aminolevulinate photodynamic therapy with cryotherapy or fluorouracil for treatment of squamous

cell carcinoma in situ: results of a multicenter randomized trial. *Arch Dermatol* 2006; **142**: 729–35.

45 Pariser DM, Lowe NJ, Stewart DM, *et al*. Photodynamic therapy with topical methyl aminolevulinate for actinic keratosis: results of a prospective randomized multicenter trial. *J Am Acad Dermatol* 2003; **48**: 227–32.

46 Szeimies RM, Matheson RT, Davis SA, *et al*. Topical methyl aminolevulinate photodynamic therapy using red light-emitting diode light for multiple actinic keratoses: a randomized study. *Dermatol Surg* 2009; **35**: 586–92.

47 Wulf HC, Philipsen P. Allergic contact dermatitis to 5-aminolaevulinic acid methylester but not to 5-aminolaevulinic acid after photodynamic therapy. *Br J Dermatol* 2004; **150**: 143–5.

48 Harries MJ, Street G, Gilmour E, Rhodes LE, Beck MH. Allergic contact dermatitis to methyl aminolevulinate (Metvix) cream used in photodynamic therapy. *Photodermatol Photoimmunol Photomed* 2007; **23**: 35–6.

49 Hohwy T, Andersen KE, Sølvsten H, Sommerlund M. Allergic contact dermatitis to methyl aminolevulinate after photodynamic therapy in 9 patients. *Contact Dermatitis* 2007; **57**: 321–3.

50 Seit S. Photodynamic photorejuvenation: an 18-month experience on combination of ALA-IPL and a 630 nm LED continuous light source. *Australas J Cosmet Surg* 2005; **1**: 26–31.

51 Zane C, Capezzera R, Sala R, Venturini M, Calzavara-Pinton P. Clinical and echographic analysis of photodynamic therapy using methylaminolevulinate as sensitizer in the treatment of photodamaged facial skin. *Lasers Surg Med* 2007; **39**: 203–9.

52 Ruiz-Rodriguez R, López-Rodriguez L. Nonablative skin resurfacing: the role of PDT. *J Drugs Dermatol* 2006; **5**: 756–62.

53 Ruiz-Rodríguez R, López L, Candelas D, Pedraz J. Photorejuvenation using topical 5-methyl aminolevulinate and red light. *J Drugs Dermatol* 2008; **7**: 633–7.

CHAPTER 6

Fillers and Botulinum Toxins

David Beynet,[1] Derek H. Jones,[1] and Timothy Corcoran Flynn[2]

[1] University of California at Los Angeles, CA, USA
[2] University of North Carolina at Chapel Hill, NC, USA

Key points

- There are a large variety of fillers now available
- Fillers can be categorized by their duration of action or actual filler material
- Botulimun toxins A have become the cosmetic toxin of choice
- Fillers and botulinum toxins are best used in conjunction with other facial rejuvenation techniques

---

Introduction

The popularity of both injectable filler substances and botulinum toxin for soft-tissue augmentation has exploded over the past two decades. These products, particularly when used in combination, can provide improvement for wrinkles and the loss of facial volume. They work synergistically as the toxin relaxes lines caused by excessive facial muscle movement, and the fillers restore lost soft-tissue mass. When combined with resurfacing of the skin, fillers and botulinum toxin may restore a youthful appearance and increase attractiveness. The focus of this chapter will be on those products with US Food and Drug Administration (FDA) clearance.

Current fillers

The use of fillers for soft tissue augmentation began over a century ago with autologous fat injection. Then, in the 1950s, liquid silicone made its debut on the cosmetic market, but was temporarily banned by the FDA until several modifications were made ensuring its purity and safety. The use of soft-tissue fillers has become more popular in recent years as hyaluronic acids (HAs) have entered the market. Bovine collagen was the gold standard of soft-tissue filling for 20 years until the first HA was approved in the USA in 2003. In the year 2007 alone, approximately 1.5 million reported

---

filler procedures were performed [1]. The US market is dominated by the HA products, with Juvederm and Restylane sharing the top sales in this market [2]. Poly-L-lactic acid, calcium hydroxyapatite, liquid injectable silicone, and human and porcine collagen are used as well, but much less frequently.

Hyaluronic acid fillers

Restylane® (Medicis, Scottsdale, AZ) is a 20 mg/cc HA filler that was FDA approved in 2003. The pivotal trial showing its safety and efficacy was performed by comparing it to Zyplast® bovine collagen (Allergan, Irvine, CA) in the contralateral nasolabial folds in each subject. This split-face study showed that Restylane provided a longer-lasting cosmetic correction and was equally well tolerated by patients. It was also shown that less injection volume was required to achieve an optimal cosmetic result. These results were noted by both patients and physicians in this double-blind study [3].

Juvederm® (Allergan, Irvine, CA) is the other commonly used HA in the USA besides Restylane and the very similar but thicker Perlane® (Medicis, Scottsdale, AZ). Juvederm and Restylane/Perlane share approximately 50% of the HA market, with others such as Elevesse and Prevelle Silk holding a smaller market share [2]. Juvederm and Restylane/Perlane are differentiated from one another, with Juvederm being a more highly cross-linked, smoother-consistency 24 mg/cc HA gel, while Restylane/Perlane is a 20 mg/cc family of granular HA gels composed of particles or beads of HA. Perlane contains larger HA beads than does Restylane and is intended for deeper and more robust volumizing. The differences between the Juvederm HA family and the Restylane/Perlane family reflect fundamental differences in processing of HA for injection after the polimerization and cross-linking of HA is completed. Proponents of Juvederm posit that compared to Restlane/Perlane, Juvederm is smoother and more cohesive after injection, although head-to-head clinical trials have yet to prove this.

Juvederm was FDA approved in 2006. As with Restylane, the pivotal trial showing the safety and efficacy of Juvederm was done comparing Juvederm (and two other similar HAs) to bovine collagen in the nasolabial folds. This split-face study showed that these smooth highly cross-linked HAs produced a clinically significant improvement of the nasolabial folds lasting 6 months or more. In addition, 88% of patients preferred the HA filler to bovine collagen. The adverse events and injection site reactions were equivalent with all fillers injected [4].

It has also been shown that after achieving optimal correction with HAs, repeat treatments lead to even longer-lasting correction than expected, with 12- to 18-month persistence of the product. This has been shown for both Juvederm and Restylane in well-designed studies [3,5] (Fig. 6.1).

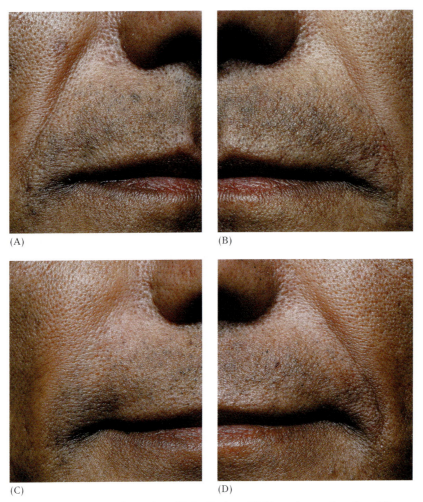

(A)   (B)

(C)   (D)

Figure 6.1 (A) Pre Juvederm Ultra. (B) Pre Zyplast. (C) 24 weeks post Juvederm Ultra (hyaluronic acid filler) to the nasolabial fold. (D) 24 weeks post Zyplast (bovine collagen) to the nasolabial fold. Photos: DHJ.

Other HA fillers on the market or soon to be on the market will be briefly discussed. Prevelle Silk® (Mentor, Santa Barbara, CA) is a 5 mg/cc HA mixed with lidocaine. It is a "softer" HA with less "lift capacity" (the so-called "G prime"), and is indicated for areas where less robust or "softer" filling is required. Its longevity is approximately 3 months, similar to human and bovine collagen. Hydrelle® (Coapt, Palo Alto, CA) is a very concentrated HA at 28 mg/cc with a higher G prime. Beletero® (Merz, Greensboro, NC) is a new HA filler not yet FDA approved in the USA. Beletero Basic is a 22.5 mg/cc HA, while Beletero Soft is a 20 mg/cc HA for more superficial filling. FDA pre-market approval is expected in 2009. Juvederm Voluma® (Allergan, Irvine, CA) is another new HA filler that is not yet FDA approved.

It is a 20 mg/cc HA of streptococcal origin with a higher lift capacity. It has a lower molecular weight and higher cross-linking ratio than other available HAs. It will be indicated for subcutaneous/supraperiosteal injection for facial volumizing and contouring.

A new trend with HA fillers is the addition of lidocaine to the product to decrease the pain of treatment. Recent studies have shown that the use of pre-incorporated lidocaine in HA fillers greatly increases patient comfort during the procedure [6].

While Juvederm and Restylane are currently sold without pre-incorporated lidocaine in the USA, these fillers are often used off-label with physician-added lidocaine, particularly for use in more sensitive areas such as the lips and periosteal locations (e.g., tear troughs). In our experience (DHJ), it is best to use a 1 : 10 dilution of 1% lidocaine with epinephrine : HA filler. The lidocaine is mixed with the filler using a female-to-female adapter with the product pushed back and forth approximately 10 times.

Another reason that HAs have become so popular is that they are, in a sense, reversible. The use of ovine testicular hyaluronidase (Vitrase®) can dissolve injected HA, which is highly useful if the product is misplaced or if there is a complication post-injection (e.g., vascular occlusion or delayed granulomatous reactions) [7]. Studies are ongoing to determine the proper dosing of hyaluronidase. In our experience (DHJ), 10 units of hyaluronidase per 0.1 cc of Juvederm or 5 units per 0.1 cc of Restylane to be dissolved is the most appropriate dose. The need for the greater amount of hyaluronidase for Juvederm is likely because the product is more highly cross-linked.

In summary, HA fillers last longer than bovine and human collagen and in general have better patient satisfaction, longer-lasting correction, and similar incidence of adverse events.

Collagen

Evolence® (Johnson & Johnson, Skilman, NJ) is cross-linked porcine collagen. It is created by taking natural porcine collagen and digesting it with pepsin to create monomeric collagen fibers. Then, accompanying immunogenic telopeptides are removed, which ultimately allows the product to be non-immunogenic. The monomeric collagen fibers are then polymerized to create reconstituted polymeric collagen. Because there are no immunogenic peptides, there is an extremely low incidence of hypersensitivity and skin testing is not required. Because of the novel mechanism of cross-linking (Glymatrix Technology), it has a longevity of up to 1 year in animal models [8].

In a pivotal trial comparing Evolence to Restylane, it was shown that the two products had similar efficacy and patient satisfaction. In this study, with 149 patients, there were no cases of hypersensitivity to the product. Bruising, swelling, and pain on injection were slightly more common with Restylane than with Evolence [8].

Evolence should not be used in the lips, as there have been reports of long-lasting (> 1 year) persistence of nodules post-injection. A "lighter" sister product, Evolence Breeze, may be more appropriate for lip injections and have a lower incidence of side effects (J. Carruthers, personal communication). This product is available in Europe and Canada, but it is not approved for use in the USA. If there is any nodularity or misplacement of Evolence, there is currently no reversing agent available, as there is for the HAs.

Calcium hydroxylapatite

Radiesse® (Bioform, Franksville, WI) is a soft-tissue filler composed of CaHA microspheres that are suspended in a carboxymethylcellulose gel. It is the third most common soft-tissue filler used currently in the USA and has been approved for the treatment of HIV lipoatrophy and for moderate to severe facial wrinkles and folds [9,10]. In histology in animal models, it has been shown that the hydroxymethylcellulose is absorbed by the tissue in approximately 6 months, while the CaHA persists and is gradually degraded by the body into calcium and phosphate ions through normal metobolic processes. It induces a robust fibroblast response that can induce collagen up to over a year.

The pivotal trial for Radiesse compared the product to human collagen for the correction of nasolabial folds. Radiesse gave significantly longer-lasting correction than to human collagen. Less total material and fewer injections were required to achieve optimal cosmetic results. The adverse-event profile of the product was similar to that of human collagen [10].

It has been compared to HAs in the Juvederm and Restylane family in a randomized trial for the treatment of nasolabial folds [11]. In this study, it was shown that CaHA ranked the highest in patient satisfaction and likelihood to return for treatment. The material was more effective and longer-lasting than the HAs in maintaining nasolabial fold augmentation. Less volume was required for full correction, and it was viewed to have a higher "lift " capacity than HA fillers (Fig. 6.2).

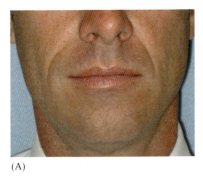
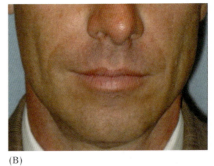

(A)   (B)

Figure 6.2 (A) Pre Radiesse. (B) Two weeks post Radiesse (calcium hydroxylapatite) to the nasolabial folds (1.3 cc). This correction persisted for about 1 year. Photos: DHJ.

Because CaHA is composed of bony material, there was concern that it could obscure reading of radiologic films. It has been shown that the volumes and densities used for facial injections do not interfere with radiographs. It is clearly visible on CT scan and minimally visible on standard x-rays, but this does not interfere with reading of films [12].

It has been shown that lidocaine can be safely added to CaHA without harmful changes in the physical properties of the original soft-tissue filler. It significantly reduces pain on injection and has become the standard of care in many practices. We recommend that lidocaine should always be added to this very robust filler, although this is considered "off-label" [13].

Radiesse is distinct from HA fillers in that it should be injected into the deep dermis or subdermal plane, whereas HA fillers are generally injected more superficially into the mid to deep dermis. It should be injected using a retrograde linear threading technique. It can be used supraperiosteally to restore volume from skeletal loss or deep mid-face volume loss. It should not be used in the lips, as nodule formation is a common complication.

A major problem that can arise from the necessity for deeper injections, as required with Radiesse, is the risk of intravascular injection or extravascular compression. Vascular compromise from either mechanism can lead to severe tissue necrosis. There have been increasing reports of angular/nasal artery occlusion with tissue necrosis secondary to injection in the superior nasolabial folds. The product should always be injected very slowly with thin linear microthreads of 0.05 cc/pass, with constant slow linear movement of the needle in the subdermal plane. Any tissue blanching should be immediately recognized and the injection stopped, and the injection site massaged, to avoid further vascular compromise. Because of increased risk of vascular compromise, Radiesse should never be used in the glabellar region. While vascular compromise can happen with any filler, it is most common with the more robust fillers. Unlike HAs, Radiesse does not have the benefit that pending necrosis can sometimes be reversed with rapid injection of hyaluronidase [7,14].

Poly-L-lactic acid

Sculptra® (Sanofi, Bridgewater, NJ) is a synthetic, resorbable, biocompatible polymer (poly-L-lactic acid) suspended in a sodium carboxymethylcellulose gel. It must be reconstituted, usually with sterile water and lidocaine 4 hours or longer in advance. This is a robust filler that must be injected into the subcutaneous plane, as superficial injections can lead to side effects including nodularity and granulomas. Collagen production is stimulated by poly-L-lactic acid (PLLA) particles, producing a gradual increase in volume over several months.

Sculptra is a good volume corrector for limited age-related lipoatrophy. The effect is subtle, and many treatments may be required to reach optimal correction, making expense a serious concern for many patients. In general,

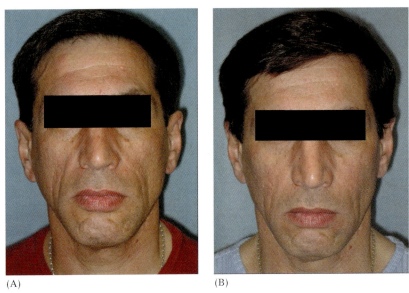

(A)   (B)

Figure 6.3 (A) Pre Sculptra for non-HIV facial lipoatrophy (age- and lean-body-mass-related). (B) One month after eight vials of Sculptra (poly-L-lactic acid; two vials injected at 1-month intervals for 4 months). Photos: DHJ.

the correction lasts longer than that achieved with many of the other fillers mentioned, usually lasting 1–2 years. This product is best used for nasolabial folds and mid-face volume enhancement. It is not appropriate for use in the lips.

Sculptra received fast-track FDA approval for treatment of HIV lipoatrophy based on four studies involving 277 patients (Sculptra Package Insert). In one study (VEGA), it was shown that with repeat treatments there was approximately a 7 mm increase in skin thickness at 1 year, as determined by ultrasound [15]. The most common adverse event was palpable sub-cutaneous nodule formation, which occurred in 52% of patients.

Overall, Sculptra is a good pan-facial volumizer, although results are subtle and a high volume of product and many treatments are needed at high cost (Fig. 6.3). Adverse events are being reported more commonly now that the product is being used more, including persistent granulo-matous reactions, which usually occur secondary to injections superficially into the dermis [16,17]. Subcutantous nodularity formation may be limited by increasing the volume of dilutent and following specific injection guide-lines recently proposed by Jones and Vleggaar [18].

Silicone

The most appropriate injectable silicone is Silikon®-1000 (Alcon, Fort Worth, TX). It is FDA approved for treatment of retinal detachment. While

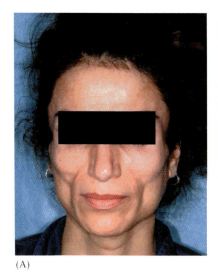
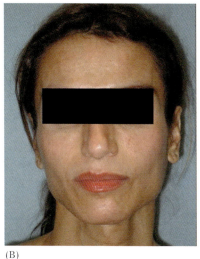

(A)   (B)

Figure 6.4 (A) Pre liquid injectable silicone for HIV-associated facial lipoatrophy.
(B) Post liquid injectable silicone (14 treatments over 2 years, 24 cc total). Photos: DHJ.

injection of Silikon-1000 for soft-tissue augmentation is legal in the USA, it
is strictly off-label. It should be injected using the microdroplet technique,
which is defined as injecting 0.01 cc per insertion into the immediate
subcutis or deeper. Limited volumes should be used at monhtly intervals. It
is our (DHJ) belief that this product is appropriate for HIV facial lipoatrophy
and acne scarring [19]. Long-term safety and efficacy remain to be proven.

In a cohort of 77 patients, injection of 2 cc/month of Silikon-1000 with the
microdroplet technique produced a consistently good correction for HIV facial
lipoatrophy. The average volume needed to get full correction was approximately 6 cc, or three treatments for each stage of lipoatrophy. Five-year safety
data on approximately 1500 patients show that there are no significant
adverse events to report at 5 years (data on file, Derek H. Jones) (Fig. 6.4).

Liquid injectable silicone has also been used with favorable results for
broad-based, depressed acne scars. At up to 30 years of follow up, patients
have shown maintenance of correction without adverse events [20]. It has
also been used to correct traumatic scars with good results.

Intradermal injection has been shown to lead to persisent visible lumps.
In general, silicone should be injected into the subcutis, except for in some
cases of acne scarring where the lift from microdroplet intradermal injection may be beneficial.

Collagen-PMMA

Polymethylmethacrylate (PMMA) suspended in bovine collagen (Artefill®;
Suneva, San Diego, CA) was FDA approved in 2006. Microscopic PMMA

particles are round, smooth, homogeneous in size and shape, and permanent. The beads stimulate collagen formation, which contributes to a long-lasting and durable correction.

The pivotal trial for Artefill compared its use to bovine collagen in the nasolabial folds. At 6 and 12 months Artefill showed continued correction while bovine collagen did not. This PMMA filler was the first soft-tissue filler to demonstrate continued improvement and persistence of correction over a 5-year period post-treatment. Of note, at 5 years 2.5% of patients had late-appearing reactions from the treatment, including lumpiness, persistent swelling or redness, or granuloma formation [21].

Newer fillers

Hydrogel polymers

While the following fillers are not FDA-approved in the US, they will be briefly mentioned here because they are available in many other countries. Bio-Alcamid® (96% water, 4% polyalkylamide) and Aquamid® (97.5% water, 2.5% polyacrylamide) are hydrogel polymers that cause fibroplasia around the periphery of these bolus-type implants. They are indicated for large volume filling, as may be required for HIV facial lipoatrophy. Infection is a major concern with these implants, with many reported late-appearing abcesses [22], which can routinely be successfully treated with antibiotics and incision and drainage of the infected implant material.

Botulinum toxins

Botulinum toxin (BTX) injection is the most common cosmetic procedure in the USA, with almost 2.8 million injections performed in 2007. This is nearly double the next most common procedure (HA injection) and five times more common than any cosmetic surgical procedure (liposuction being the most common) [1]. The FDA approved Botox® (Allergan Inc., Irvine, CA) in 1989 for the treatment of specific ocular disorders. In patients receiving BTX treatments for blepharospasm, wrinkles were reduced. This led to its cosmetic approval for the treatment of glabellar lines in 2002. The use of BTX has been clearly shown to be the leader in non-invasive treatment of glabellar, forehead, and periocular dynamic rhytides. Its cosmetic use has continued to expand to treat many other areas including the midface, perioral area, and neck. It can also be combined with other treatment modalities such as laser resurfacing and fillers, which can lead to enhanced aesthetic outcomes (Figs. 6.5, 6.6).

BTXs are produced by strains of the bacteria *Clostridium botulinum* and are some of the most potent neurotoxins known, with lethal doses of just

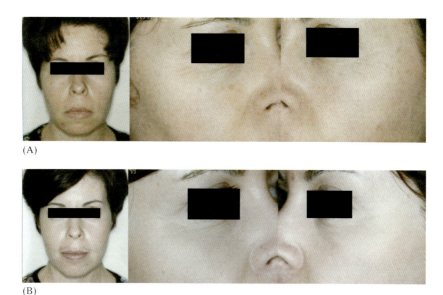

(A)

(B)

Figure 6.5 (A) Pre BOTOX and CO_2 laser resurfacing. (B) Post BOTOX and CO_2 laser resurfacing. Photos: DHJ.

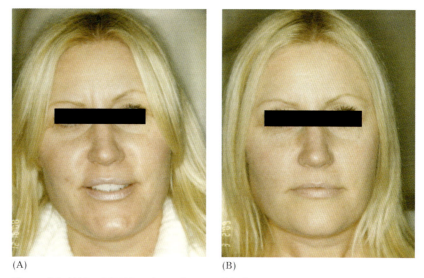

(A)   (B)

Figure 6.6 (A) Pre BOTOX and Juvederm to glabella. (B) Post BOTOX and Juvederm to glabella. Photos: DHJ.

10^{-9} g/kg body weight [23]. There are seven known serotypes of botulinum toxin, types A through G. They all act by inhibiting the release of acetylcholine at the presynaptic terminal of the neuromuscular junction. Serotypes A, C, and E catalyze the cleavage of SNAP-25, while B, D, F, and G catalyze the cleavage of synatobrevin (VAMP). Both SNAP-25 and synaptobrevin are part of the SNARE complex of proteins necessary for presynaptic vesicular release of acetylcholine. The cleavage of these proteins causes chemodenervation of the targeted muscles for approximately 3–4 months. Ultimately, muscle activity returns due to natural recovery of the neuromuscular junction.

Side effects of BTX injection are usually minimal with proper dosing and injection technique. Inadvertent paralysis of non-targeted muscles or glandular tissue can result in eyelid ptosis, diplopia, difficulty closing the eyes, decreased tearing, inability to pucker the lips, weakness while chewing, and others. Targeted injection with concentrated product can help to avoid these complications [24].

Contraindications to the use of Botox (which here we assume to include all BTXs) include diseases which affect the neuromuscular junction, pregnancy, and lactation. Patients with myasthenia gravis and Lambert–Eaton thus should not be treated. While no adverse events have been reported with Botox injection during pregnancy, it is classified as pregnancy category C and should not be used for cosmetic purposes in this setting. Medications such as aminoglycosides, penicillamine, quinine, and calcium channel blockers can also affect the neuromuscular junction, and BTX should therefore not be used in patients taking these medications [24].

Resistance

Resistance to BTX has been well documented [25,26], but rarely in the cosmetic setting. In general, it occurs after repeated injections of high doses (> 100 units per treatment). Resistance to one serotype of BTX does not usually cause resistance to the other serotypes. For example, a patient who becomes resistant to BTX-A will most likely still respond to BTX-B. However, this can still be a problem as certain serotypes have been proven to be more effective for treatment than others.

Resistance is thought to develop to the complexing proteins which are used to stabilize the product, not to the toxin itself. Manufacturers are therefore aiming to develop BTX with as few stabilizing proteins as possible (e.g., the Mentor Corporation and Merz, which have developed PurTox® and Xeomin®, respectively).

Injection technique

Tuberculin or insulin syringes are commonly used for BTX injection. In particular insulin syringes are preferred, as they may waste less product, having no dead space in the hub. Most frequently used is the 0.3 cc Ultra-Fine® II 31 g insulin syringe [27]. Topical analgesia is not required, but using ice may reduce pain and constrict blood vessels, thereby lessening the chance of bruising.

Patients should be positioned sitting upright or near upright, as the effects of gravity do affect the appearance of the areas to be treated. The patient should be asked to contract and relax sequentially the muscles in the area to be treated. In this way, the physician can determine where the underlying musculature is situated and any baseline asymmetries.

Facial aesthetic enhancement with BTX is an art, and no two patients should necessarily be treated exactly the same. Evaluating the patient at full contraction and relaxation, and with background knowledge of the facial musculature in mind, appropriate treatment can be determined. General differences to keep in mind during treatment are that men in general require higher doses per treatment area, and that thin muscles such as the platysma require much lower doses than larger muscles such as the corrugators. Baseline muscular variations should also be kept in mind. For example, certain patients (commonly Asians and the elderly) may present with unique brow or lid position at baseline, and the treatment patterns and doses of BTX utilized should minimize the chance of causing an undesirable result.

Review of botulinum toxins

Although Botox Cosmetic® (Allergan, Irvine, CA) and Dysport® (Ipsen, UK; Medicis, Scottsdale, AZ) are the only FDA-approved BTXs for cosmetic use in the USA, there are many other toxins available for cosmetic use in other countries, and some of these will likely be approved in the USA. These BTXs will be discussed below (Table 6.1).

Botox Cosmetic/Vistabel/Vistabex (Allergan Inc.)

Botox Cosmetic (marketed as Vistabel® in the United Kingdom and Vistabex® in Italy) is the original BTX type-A product. It has been the most studied and widely used BTX. Consistent results and a low side-effect profile are characteristic. The only modification of the original toxin occurred in 1997, when the amount of immunogenic protein in the product was reduced. Botox currently represents 85% of the world market for BTX [29].

Botox Cosmetic is supplied as a vacuum-dried powder, 100 units per vial. Unreconstituted Botox Cosmetic should be stored at 2–8 °C. The manufacturer's recommendation is to reconstitute the Botox with 2.5 mL of 0.9% non-preserved saline to a final concentration of 4.0 U/0.1 mL. Decreased pain of injection has been shown with the use of preserved saline [30]. With proper storage at 4 °C (never frozen), the reconstituted product can be stored for up to 6 weeks without loss of potency.

Dysport (Medicis and Ipsen)

Dysport®, manufactured by Ipsen (distributed in the US by Medicis), is another BTX-A product with the same mechanism of action as Botox. It received FDA pre-market approval in April 2009. The Dysport protein is produced through a column separation technique, while Botox is produced through repeated precipitation and redissolution methods.

Table 6.1 Summary of botulinum toxin products approved or under development for cosmetic indications. Reproduced from Carruthers and Carruthers [28] with permission from Skincareguide.com.

	Botox®	Botox® Cosmetic/Vistabel®/Vistabex®	Dysport®/Reloxin®	Dysport® Cosmetic	Myobloc®/NeuroBloc®	NT-201/XEOMIN®	PurTox®
Company	Allergan Inc.	Allergan Inc.	Ipsen Inc./Medicis Inc.	Ipsen Inc./Medicis Inc.	Solstice Neurosciences Inc.	Merz Pharmaceuticals	Mentor Corporation
Type	Type A, Hall strain	Type A, Hall strain	Type A	Type A	Type B	Type A, Hall strain	Type A, Hall strain
Approvals	In over 75 countries worldwide, including US and Canada	In over 16 countries, including US, Canada, Italy, France	In over 65 countries; not approved in US or Canada	Germany, other European countries	Some European countries, US, Canada	Germany, other European countries, Mexico, Argentina	None
Active substance (molecular weight)	Botulinum toxin type A complex (900 kD)	Botulinum toxin type A complex (900 kD)	Botulinum toxin type A complex (900 kD)*	Botulinum toxin type A complex (900 kD)*	Botulinum toxin type B complex (700 kD)	Botulinum toxin type A, free from complexing proteins (150 kD)	Botulinum toxin type A, free from complexing proteins (150 kD)
Strength of action (BTX-A:Product)	1:1	1:1	1:2–1:4 (approximate)	1:2–1:4 (approximate)	1:50–1:100	1:1	1:1.5 ?
Indications	Blepharospasm; cervical dystonia; glabellar lines; hyperhidrosis	Glabellar lines	Blepharospasm; cervical dystonia	Glabellar lines	Cervical dystonia	Blepharospasm; cervical dystonia; glabellar lines in Argentina	Phase 3 for glabellar lines; Phase 1 for spasmodic torticollis/cervical dystonia

Mode of action	SNAP-25	SNAP-25	SNAP-25	SNAP-25	VAMP	SNAP-25	SNAP-25
Pharmaceutical form	Powder dissolved in solution for injection	Powder dissolved in solution for injection	Powder dissolved in solution for injection	Powder dissolved in solution for injection	Solution	Powder dissolved in solution for injection	Powder dissolved in solution for injection
Units/vial	100	50	500	300 or 500	2500; 5000; 10 000	100	?
Volume	10 mL maximum	1.25 mL or 2.5 mL recommended	2.5 mL recommended	5 mL maximum	0.5 mL; 1 mL; 2 mL	8 mL maximum	?
Reconstitution	0.9% NaCl solution	0.9% NaCl solution	0.9% NaCl solution	0.9% NaCl solution	Prepared solution, dilutable	0.9% NaCl solution	0.9% NaCl solution
Storage	2–8 °C or <–5 °C	2–8 °C or <–5 °C	2–8 °C	2–8 °C	2–8 °C do not freeze	Up to 25 °C	?

SNAP-25 (synaptosomal associated protein with the molecular mass of 25 kD), an intracellular protein that is essential for synaptic vesicle transmission; it has been identified as the molecular target of BTX-A.

VAMP (synaptobrevin), a protein involved in synaptic vesicle movement that has been identified as the molecular target of BTX-B.

* The formulation contains complexes of variable size between 500 and 900 kD.

? Data unavailable or unconfirmed.

Studies comparing Botox to Dysport are difficult as there has been no clear determination of comparable dosages of the two products. However, in the largest double-blind, randomized, parallel-group study comparing the efficacy and side-effect profile of Botox versus Dysport in the glabellar lines of 62 patients, it was noted that Botox had a longer duration of action with a similar side-effect profile [31]. Dysport has been extensively studied in the glabellar complex, with doses of 50 units being used in the clinical trials [32].

PurTox (Mentor Corporation)
PurTox® is an uncomplexed BTX-A product developed to decrease the amount of complexed protein with botulinum toxin in hopes to decrease immunogenic resistance. As mentioned earlier, increased amount of non-toxin protein injected is thought to increase the development of resistance to BTX. PurTox is currently in phase III trials for cosmetic use in the USA. It is stable at room temperature, unlike Botox or Dysport.

NT-201/Xeomin (Merz Pharmaceuticals)
Xeomin®, also known as NT 201, is a BTX-A free of complexing proteins. While Botox and Dysport have protein counts of 5 mg per vial, Xeomin has just 0.6 mg/vial. It is approved for use in Germany and 11 other European countries, Canada, Argentina, and Mexico [33].

In the past, complexing proteins have been thought to influence diffusion. However, Kerscher *et al.* studied the diffusion of Xeomin and did a direct comparison to Botox in 20 patients. The forehead was used as the site, and equal amounts of Botox and Xeomin were injected. Forehead lines were studied, and the anhydrotic areas compared. The products were comparable [34].

Myobloc/NeuroBloc (Solstice Neurosciences Inc.; Eisai Co. Ltd.)
Myobloc® is currently the only BTX-B product that is available on the market. It is approved for cervical dystonia in North America. It has an acidic pH of ~5.5, which can make injections more painful than other BTXs. In studies of Myobloc for cosmetic purposes, it has been shown to have a quicker onset of action compared to BTX-A products, but it does not appear to last as long. It also has a greater area of diffusion [35–38]. It can be used for patients who desire a rapid onset of action. It has also been used by one of us (TCF) to treat patients who are not satisfied with the results of the type A toxin. The increased diffusion of the toxin must be borne in mind when selecting injection points.

CBTX-A/Chinatox/Prosigne® (Lanzhou Institute of Biological Products)
Chinatox is the only approved BTX-A in the People's Republic of China. Instead of using human serum albumin as the complexing protein (like

Botox and Dysport), Chinatox uses a bovine gelatin protein. This leads to increased sensitization, occasional skin rashes, and in some cases bovine spongiform encephalopathy [28]. There are few scientific studies on this product.

Neuronox (Medy-Tox Inc.)

Neuronox® is a BTX-A product and is approved for medical uses in Korea and South America. It is widely used in Korea and Southeast Asia for cosmetic purposes. It appears to have similar unit dosing and efficacy to Botox [39]. Few studies exist.

Conclusion

In summary, fillers and botulinum toxins have proven to be a very effective and safe treatment for dynamic facial rhytides and other cosmetic concerns for over 20 years. These products are relatively easy to administer if proper training has been completed and the provider has a good understanding of the facial musculature.

There are now a large variety of fillers available both in the USA and around the world. Botox has the highest number of peer-reviewed studies proving its efficacy and safety. However, there are many BTXs available in other countries and many that are in clinical trials that may be soon available for use in the USA. As these toxins are further developed and new variations arise, we will have a better understanding of which toxins are the safest and most efficacious.

References

1 American Society for Aesthetic Plastic Surgery. Cosmetic procedures in 2007. www.miinews.com (accessed April 14, 2009).

3 Narins RS, Dayan SH, Brandt FS, Baldwin EK. Persistence and improvement of nasolabial fold correction with nonanimal-stabilized hyaluronic acid 100 000 gel particles/mL filler on two retreatment schedules: results up to 18 months on two retreatment schedules. *Dermatol Surg* 2008; **34**: S2–8.

4 Baumann LS, Shamban AT, Lupo MP, *et al.* Comparison of smooth-gel hyaluronic acid dermal fillers with cross-linked bovine collagen: a multicenter, double-masked, randomized, within-subject study. *Dermatol Surg* 2007; **33**: S128–35.

5 Smith S, Jones D. Efficacy and safety following repeat treatment for a new family of hyaluronic acid based fillers. Poster presentation, American Academy of Dermatology Academy 2006 Meeting. San Diego, CA, 2006.

6 Levy PM, De Boulle K, Raspaldo H. Comparison of injection comfort of a new category of cohesive hyaluronic acid filler with preincorporated lidocaine and a hyaluronic acid filler alone. *Dermatol Surg* 2009; **35** (Suppl. 1): 332–6.

7 Brody HJ. Use of hyaluronidase in the treatment of granulomatous hyaluronic acid reactions or unwanted hyaluronic acid misplacement. *Dermatol Surg* 2005; **31**: 893–7.

8 Narins RS, Brandt FS, Lorenc ZP, Maas CS, Monheit GD, Smith SR. Twelve-month persistency of a novel ribose-cross-linked collagen dermal filler. *Dermatol Surg* 2008; **34**: S31–9.

9 Carruthers A, Carruthers J. Evaluation of injectable calcium hydroxylapatite for the treatment of facial lipoatrophy associated with human immunodeficiency virus. *Dermatol Surg* 2008; **34**: 1486–99.

10 Smith S, Busso M, McClaren M, Bass LS. A randomized, bilateral, prospective comparison of calcium hydroxylapatite microspheres versus human-based collagen for the correction of nasolabial folds. *Dermatol Surg* 2007; **33**: S112–21.

11 Moers-Carpi MM, Tufet JO. Calcium hydroxylapatite versus nonanimal stabilized hyaluronic acid for the correction of nasolabial folds: a 12-month, multicenter, prospective, randomized, controlled, split-face trial. *Dermatol Surg* 2008; **34**: 210–15.

12 Carruthers A, Liebeskind M, Carruthers J, Forster BB. Radiographic and computed tomographic studies of calcium hydroxylapatite for treatment of HIV-associated facial lipoatrophy and correction of nasolabial folds. *Dermatol Surg* 2008; **34**: S78–84.

13 Busso M, Voigts R. An investigation of changes in physical properties of injectable calcium hydroxylapatite in a carrier gel when mixed with lidocaine and with lidocaine/epinephrine. *Dermatol Surg* 2008; **34**: S16–23.

14 Hirsch RJ, Cohen JL, Carruthers JD. Successful management of an unusual presentation of impending necrosis following a hyaluronic acid injection embolus and a proposed algorithm for management with hyaluronidase. *Dermatol Surg* 2007; **33**: 357–60.

15 Valantin MA, Aubron-Olivier C, Ghosn J, *et al.* Polylactic acid implants (New-Fill) to correct facial lipoatrophy in HIV-infected patients: results of the open-label study VEGA. *AIDS* 2003; **17**: 2471–7.

16 Stewart DB, Morganroth GS, Mooney MA, Cohen J, Levin PS, Gladstone HB. Management of visible granulomas following periorbital injection of poly-L-lactic Acid. *Ophthal Plast Reconstr Surg* 2007; **23**: 298–301.

17 Wildemore JK, Jones DH. Persistent granulomatous inflammatory response induced by injectable poly-L-lactic acid for HIV lipoatrophy. *Dermatol Surg* 2006; **32**: 1407–9.

18 Jones DH, Vleggaar D. Technique for injecting poly-L-lactic acid. *J Drugs Dermatol* 2007; **6**: S13–17.

19 Jones DH, Carruthers A, Orentreich D, *et al.* Highly purified 1000-cSt silicone oil for treatment of human immunodeficiency virus-associated facial lipoatrophy: an open pilot trial. *Dermatol Surg* 2004; **30**: 1279–86.

20 Barnett JG, Barnett CR. Treatment of acne scars with liquid silicone injections: 30-year perspective. *Dermatol Surg* 2005; **31**: 1542–9.

21 Carruthers A, Carruthers JD. Polymethylmethacrylate microspheres/collagen as a tissue augmenting agent: personal experience over 5 years. *Dermatol Surg* 2005; **31**: 1561–4.

22 Jones DH, Carruthers A, Fitzgerald R, Sarantopoulos GP, Binder S. Late-appearing abscesses after injections of nonabsorbable hydrogel polymer for HIV-associated facial lipoatrophy. *Dermatol Surg* 2007; **33**: S193–8.

23 Lamanna C. The most poisonous poison. *Science* 1959; **130**: 763–72.

24 Klein AW. Contraindications and complications with the use of botulinum toxin. *Clin Dermatol* 2004; **22**: 66–75.

25 Borodic G. Immunologic resistance after repeated botulinum toxin type a injections for facial rhytides. *Ophthal Plast Reconstr Surg* 2006; **22**: 239–40.

26 Borodic G, Johnson E, Goodnough M, Schantz E. Botulinum toxin therapy, immunologic resistance, and problems with available materials. *Neurology* 1996; **46**: 26–9.

27 Flynn TC, Carruthers A, Carruthers J. Surgical pearl: the use of the Ultra-Fine II short needle 0.3-cc insulin syringe for botulinum toxin injections. *J Am Acad Dermatol* 2002; **46**: 931–3.

28 Carruthers A, Carruthers J. Botulinum toxin products overview. *Skin Therapy Lett* 2008; **13**: 1–4.

29 Carruthers J, Carruthers A. The evolution of botulinum neurotoxin type A for cosmetic applications. *J Cosmet Laser Ther* 2007; **9**: 186–92.

30 Alam M, Dover JS, Arndt KA. Pain associated with injection of botulinum A exotoxin reconstituted using isotonic sodium chloride with and without preservative: a double-blind, randomized controlled trial. *Arch Dermatol* 2002; **138**: 510–14.

31 Lowe P, Patnaik R, Lowe N. Comparison of two formulations of botulinum toxin type A for the treatment of glabellar lines: a double-blind, randomized study. *J Am Acad Dermatol* 2006; **55**: 975–80.

32 Rzany B, Ascher B, Fratila A, Monheit GD, Talarico S, Sterry W. Efficacy and safety of 3- and 5-injection patterns (30 and 50 U) of botulinum toxin A (Dysport) for the treatment of wrinkles in the glabella and the central forehead region. *Arch Dermatol* 2006; **142**: 320–6.

33 Xeomin.com. www.xeomin.com (accessed April 14, 2009).

34 Kerscher M, Maack M, Reuther T, Krueger N. Diffusion characteristics of two different neurotoxins in patients with symmetric forehead lines. *J Am Acad Dermatol* 2007; **56** (Suppl. 2): AB199.

35 Jacob CI. Botulinum neurotoxin type B: a rapid wrinkle reducer. *Semin Cutan Med Surg* 2003; **22**: 131–5.

36 Spencer JM. Botulinum toxin B: the new option in cosmetic injection. *J Drugs Dermatol* 2002; **1**: 17–22.

37 Spencer JM, Gordon M, Goldberg DJ. Botulinum B treatment of the glabellar and frontalis regions: a dose response analysis. *J Cosmet Laser Ther* 2002; **4**: 19–23.

38 Flynn TC, Clark RE. Botulinum toxin type B (MYOBLOC) versus botulinum toxin type A (BOTOX) frontalis study: rate of onset and radius of diffusion. *Dermatol Surg* 2003; **29**: 519–22.

39 Stone AV, Ma J, Whitlock PW, *et al.* Effects of Botox and Neuronox on muscle force generation in mice. *J Orthop Res* 2007; **25**: 1658–64.

CHAPTER 7

Cosmeceuticals

Zoe Diana Draelos
New Jersey Medical School, Newark, New Jersey, USA

Key points

- Cosmeceuticals can be complementary to facial resurfacing procedures
- Moisturizers can decrease transepidermal water loss
- Hyperpigmentation induced by facial resurfacing can be prevented or decreased with cosmeceuticals
- Antioxidants, in the form of polyphenols and flavonoids, can enhance skin appearance

---

Introduction

Cosmeceuticals can be complementary to facial resurfacing procedures by promoting healing, minimizing post-inflammatory hyperpigmentation, and maintaining the desired result. Even though cosmeceuticals are over-the-counter (OTC) preparations, they cannot be overlooked in the post-resurfacing healing period and should be discussed when recommending a skin-care maintenance regimen following resurfacing. Moisturizers can decrease transepidermal water loss from freshly wounded skin, providing pain control and speeding barrier repair. The most common adverse event from facial resurfacing is undesirable pigmentation, which can be prevented or decreased with substances that inhibit a key step in the melanin synthetic pathway. Finally, antioxidants, in the form of polyphenols and flavonoids, can enhance skin appearance when combined with moisturization. This chapter discusses the use of cosmeceuticals relevant to facial resurfacing.

Moisturizers

The main cutaneous function of cosmeceuticals is to enhance the barrier function of the skin following a resurfacing procedure. Enhancing the barrier decreases stinging and burning from a sensory standpoint and improves the look and feel of the skin. Moisturizers can smooth down

---

Facial Resurfacing, 1st edition. Edited by David J. Goldberg. © 2010 Blackwell Publishing.

desquamating corneocytes and fill in the gaps between the remaining corneocytes to create the impression of tactile smoothness. This effect is temporary, of course, until the moisturizer is removed from the skin surface by wiping or cleansing. From a functional standpoint, moisturizers can create an optimal environment for healing and minimize the appearance of lines of dehydration by decreasing transepidermal water loss. Transepidermal water loss increases when the brick-and-mortar organization of the protein-rich corneocytes held together by intercellular lipids is damaged. A well-formulated cosmeceutical moisturizer can decrease the water loss until healing occurs following a resurfacing procedure.

There are two cosmeceutical ingredient categories that can reduce transepidermal water loss post-resurfacing: occlusives and humectants [1]. The most common method for reducing transepidermal water loss is the application of occlusive ingredients in combination with humectant ingredients in a thin moisturizer film.

Occlusive moisturizers

Occlusive moisturizers contain oily substances that create a barrier to water evaporation. The more commonly used occlusive ingredients in current formulations and their chemical category are listed in Table 7.1 [2]. The most popular and effective occlusive ingredient used following resurfacing is petrolatum. Petrolatum is effective because it blocks 99% of water loss from the skin surface [3]. This remaining 1% transepidermal water loss is necessary to provide the cellular message for barrier repair initiation following wounding. If the transepidermal water loss is completely halted, the removal of the occlusion results in failure to repair the barrier, and water loss quickly resumes at its pre-application level. Thus the occlusion does not initiate barrier repair [4]. Petrolatum does not function as an impermeable barrier, rather it permeates throughout the interstices of the stratum corneum, allowing barrier function to be re-established [5].

Table 7.1 Moisturizing ingredients for barrier enhancement.

1 Hydrocarbon oils and waxes: petrolatum, mineral oil, paraffin, squalene
2 Silicone oils
3 Vegetable and animal fats
4 Fatty acids: lanolin acid, stearic acid
5 Fatty alcohol: lanolin alcohol, cetyl alcohol
6 Polyhydric alcohols: propylene glycol
7 Wax esters: lanolin, beeswax, stearyl stearate
8 Vegetable waxes: carnauba, candelilla
9 Phospholipids: lecithin
10 Sterols: cholesterol

Humectant moisturizers

Another concept in rehydrating the stratum corneum is the use of humectants. Humectants have been used in cosmetics for many years to increase shelf life by preventing product evaporation and subsequent thickening due to variations in temperature and humidity. Humectants are a necessary in all oil-in-water creams to maintain the required water content. Substances that function as humectants include glycerin, honey, sodium lactate, urea, propylene glycol, sorbitol, pyrrolidone carboxylic acid, gelatin, hyaluronic acid, vitamins, and some proteins [3,6].

Following resurfacing, the barrier has been injured, and water must be drawn to the wounded skin to prevent desiccation, which slows healing. Desiccation of the facial skin also leads to an undesirable sensation of pulling and drawing. Humectants attract water from the deeper epidermal and dermal tissues to rehydrate the stratum corneum. This water is trapped by the occlusive moisturizing ingredients in a thin film on top of the stratum corneum [7]. Humectants may also allow the skin to feel smoother by filling holes in the stratum corneum through swelling [8,9]. Therefore, a good moisturizer should combine both occlusive and humectant ingredients.

There is no doubt that most anti-aging cosmeceuticals are primarily well-constructed moisturizers containing occlusive and humectant ingredients. Furthermore, most of the claims associated with cosmeceuticals are moisturizer claims. Keep in mind that the moisturizer is really the vehicle for transporting the special ingredient to the skin surface, but the vehicle may actually be the active ingredient in many cosmeceutical formulations. Thus, cosmeceuticals can be used to aid healing and maintain an excellent result following skin resurfacing.

Pigment lightening agents

Post-inflammatory hyperpigmentation is the most common adverse side effect of facial resurfacing. The best treatment for this unwanted pigmentation is prevention in the form of adequate photoprotection. Beyond photoprotection, there are a variety of cosmeceutical ingredients that can interrupt melanin formation. However, cosmeceutical treatments for hyperpigmentation are problematic. A successful treatment must remove existing pigment from the skin, shut down the manufacture of melanin, and prevent the transfer of existing melanin to the melanosomes.

Many cosmetic products are available to lighten skin and improve even skin tone. These products typically do not contain hydroquinone, but rather other botanically derived products that interrupt melanin synthesis. These botanicals include ascorbic acid, licorice extract, alpha-lipoic acid, kojic acid, aleosin, and arbutin. Hydroquinone has been eliminated from most cosmetics, since the European Union and Asia have removed hydroquinone from the OTC market. Most cosmetics companies are international in their distribution and formulate for the global market and not specifically for the United States market, where OTC hydroquinone is still allowed. This discussion evaluates ingredients to prevent skin darkening following facial resurfacing.

Photoprotection

Many new developments have occurred in the photoprotection cosmeceutical market to increase both efficacy and cosmetic acceptability. Higher sun protection factor (SPF) formulations are more popular as new sunscreen combinations arise that provide better ultraviolet B (UVB) protection. New methods of increasing the longevity of UVA photoprotectants provide better broad-spectrum protection. These advances have improved the ability of sunscreens to prevent post-inflammatory hyperpigmentation following resurfacing.

Sunscreen filters can be classified into two major categories, chemical and physical. Chemical sunscreens, also known as organic filters, undergo a chemical transformation, known as resonance delocalization, to absorb UV radiation and transform it to heat. This reaction occurs within the phenol ring, which contains an electron-releasing group in the ortho and/or para position, and is irreversible, rendering the sunscreen inactive once it has absorbed the UV radiation. Physical sunscreens, also known as inorganic filters, are usually ground particulates that reflect or scatter UV radiation, absorbing relatively little of the energy. For this reason they have longer activity on the skin surface.

The most important protection following facial resurfacing is from UVA radiation, which is directly responsible for pigment production. Two important UVA filters include oxybenzone and avobenzone. Oxybenzone provides weak UVA photoprotection below 320 nm. It is commonly combined with avobenzone (Parsol 1789®). Unfortunately, avobenzone is highly photounstable, with 36% of the avobenzone destroyed shortly after sun exposure. It is estimated that all of the avobenzone is gone from a sunscreen after 5 hours or 50 joules of exposure, necessitating frequent reapplication. Avobenzone is also chemically incompatible with other commonly used inorganic filters, such as zinc oxide and titanium dioxide. However, avobenzone has assumed new importance in a proprietary sunscreen complex, known as Helioplex® (Neutrogena), combining avobenzone with oxybenzone and Hallbrite® TQ to create a photostable avobenzone with long-lasting UVA photoprotectant qualities. Hallbrite TQ is chemically known as 2-6-diethylhexylnaphthalate. Photostable UVA organic filters are important cosmeceuticals following resurfacing.

Another important UVA photoprotection in facial resurfacing is ecam-sule, better known as Mexoryl®. Mexoryl (L'Oreal) was originally developed to stabilize avobenzone. It is used in combination with oxybenzone and octocrylene to provide excellent protection from post-inflammatory hyper-pigmentation following resurfacing. It is available in two forms: Mexoryl SX and Mexoryl XL. Mexoryl SX is a water-soluble form that is suitable for daywear sunscreen formulations. This would include sunscreen-containing moisturizers, sunscreens, and cosmeceuticals. Mexoryl XL is an oil-soluble form that is suitable for water-resistant sunscreen formulations, including those worn on the beach and during vigorous physical exercise. Only Mexoryl SX has been approved for use in the USA.

The inorganic UVA/UVB filters titanium dioxide and zinc oxide are also important in preventing post-inflammatory hyperpigmentation following resurfacing. Titanium dioxide is usually micronized to contain particles of many sizes to provide optimal UV scattering abilities. Unfortunately, it leaves a white film on the skin and is used mainly for beachwear sunscreens and not cosmeceuticals. Zinc oxide is usually available in a microfine form, meaning it contains small particles of one size, making it appropriate for day wear. A newly introduced colorless zinc oxide with extremely small particles is finding its way into many post-resurfacing cosmeceuticals, but there is concern that the nanoparticles may enter the skin through appendageal structures, creating a permanent reservoir. The cosmeceutical industry has placed a voluntary hold on nanoparticle inorganic filters and pigments until the penetration issues are better understood.

Ascorbic acid

Ascorbic acid, also known as vitamin C, is used in cosmeceuticals for the treatment and prevention of hyperpigmentation because it interrupts melanogenesis by interacting with copper ions to reduce dopaquinone and block dihydrochinindol-2-carboxyl acid oxidation [10]. Ascorbic acid, an antioxidant, is rapidly oxidized when exposed to air, with limited stability. For this reason, many cosmeceuticals are using the more stable magnesium ascorbyl phosphate, which is metabolized to ascorbic acid in the skin. High concentrations of ascorbic acid must be used with caution, however, as the low pH can be irritating to the skin. Pigment-lightening cosmeceuticals may contain ascorbic acid as a pH adjustor or to function as an antioxidant preservative. It is important to recognize that ascorbic acid is a multifunc-tional ingredient with very minimal pigment-lightening capabilities.

Licorice extract

Licorice extracts are found in cosmeceuticals to decrease facial redness and reduce pigmentation. The extract contains liquiritin and isoliquertin, which are glycosides containing flavenoids [11], which induce skin lightening by dispersing melanin. To see clinical results, the liquiritin must be applied in the dose of 1 g per day for 4 weeks. Irritation is not a side effect, as is so frequently observed with hydroquinone and ascorbic acid, but efficacy is minimal.

Alpha-lipoic acid

Alpha-lipoic acid is found in a variety of anti-aging cosmeceuticals to function as an antioxidant [12], but it may also have very limited pigment-lightening properties. It is a disulfide derivative of octanoic acid that is able to inhibit tyrosinase. However, it is a large molecule and cutaneous penetration to the level of the melanocyte is challenging, significantly reducing its efficacy.

Kojic acid

Kojic acid, chemically known as 5-hydroxymethyl-4H-pyrane-4-one, is one of the most popular cosmeceutical skin-lightening agents found in cosmetic-counter skin-lightening creams distributed worldwide. It is a hydrophilic fungal derivative obtained from *Aspergillus* and *Penicillium* species. It is the agent most commonly employed in East Asia for the treatment of melasma, but it is highly unstable [13]. Newer formulations have incorporated kojic dipalmitate, but the efficacy of this derivative has not been well studied. Some research indicates that kojic acid is equivalent to hydroquinone in pigment-lightening ability [14]. The activity of kojic acid is attributed to its ability to prevent tyrosinase activity by binding to copper.

Aleosin

Aleosin is a low-molecular-weight glycoprotein obtained from the aloe vera plant. It is a natural hydroxymethylchromone functioning to inhibit tyrosinase by competitive inhibition at the DOPA oxidation site [15,16]. In contrast to hydroquinone, it shows no cell cytotoxicity, but it has limited ability to penetrate the skin due to its hydrophilic nature. The effects of aleosin have been largely demonstrated in pigmented skin equivalents, not human-use studies [17]. It is sometimes mixed with arbutin to enhance its skin-lightening abilities.

Arbutin

Arbutin, chemically known as 4-hydroxyphenyl-beta-glucopyranoside, is obtained from the leaves of the *Vaccinium vitis-idaea* and other related plants. It is a naturally occurring gluconopyranoside that causes decreased tyrosinase activity without affecting messenger RNA expression [18]. It also inhibits melanosome maturation. Arbutin is not toxic to melanocytes and is used in a variety of pigment-lightening preparations in Japan at concentrations of 3%. Higher concentrations are more efficacious than lower concentrations, but a paradoxical pigment darkening may occur. Arbutin-beta-glycosides have been produced that are less cytotoxic than arbutin [19].

Hydroquinone

The gold standard for the treatment of hyperpigmentation in the USA remains hydroquinone. This substance is actually quite controversial, having been removed from the OTC markets in Europe and Asia. Concern arose because oral hydroquinone has been reported to cause cancer in mice fed large amounts of the substance. While oral consumption probably is not related to topical application, hydroquinone remains controversial because it is toxic to melanocytes. Hydroquinone, a phenolic compound chemically known as 1,4-dihydroxybenzene, functions by inhibiting the enzymatic oxidation of tyrosine and phenol oxidases. It covalently binds to histidine or interacts with copper at the active site of tyrosinase. It also inhibits RNA and DNA synthesis and may alter melanosome formation, thus selectively damaging melanocytes. These activities suppress the melanocyte metabolic processes, inducing gradual decrease of melanin pigment production [20]. Hydroquinone is still the best option for lightening post-inflammatory hyperpigmentation following resurfacing.

Antioxidants

Antioxidants form one of the most popular categories of cosmeceutical ingredients. This is due to the fact that the major cause of cutaneous aging is oxidation of skin structures from highly reactive oxygen molecules present in our oxygen-rich environment. It is amazing to think that the life-giving oxygen required to survive is also the same oxygen responsible for aging the human body. The primary source of cosmeceutical antioxidant ingredients is botanical extracts, since all plants must protect themselves from oxidation following UV exposure.

Antioxidant botanicals function by quenching singlet oxygen and reactive oxygen species, such as superoxide anions, hydroxyl radicals, fatty peroxy radicals, and hydroperoxides. There are many botanical antioxidants available, both from raw-material suppliers and from the cosmeceutical industry, and they can be classified in three categories, carotenoids, flavonoids, and polyphenols. Carotenoids are chemically related to retinoids, while flavonoids possess a polyphenolic structure that accounts for their antioxidant, UV-protectant, and metal chelation abilities. Lastly, polyphenols represent a chemical subset of flavonoids.

Antioxidants are found in many skin lines for use following resurfacing procedures. They are typically placed in moisturizing vehicles that may aid in healing through the prevention of transepidermal water loss. Whether the antioxidant formulation extends the effect of a resurfacing procedure has never been documented, yet their frequent use demands a thorough understanding of their function.

Carotenoids

Carotenoids are derivatives of vitamin A and have found widespread use in cosmeceuticals due to the established topical anti-aging benefits associated with the prescription retinoid tretinoin. The carotenoids are a large family of orange, red, and yellow substances that perform vital antioxidant roles when ingested and are less well established as topical antioxidants. The carotenoids are discussed in detail here.

Astaxanthin

Astaxanthin is a pink carotenoid found in high concentration in salmon, accounting for the characteristic pink color of the fish. This is the rationale for anti-aging diets recommending the ingestion of a serving of salmon five times weekly [21]. For topical application purposes, astaxanthin is obtained from the marine microalgae *Haematococcus pluvialis*. The efficacy of astaxanthin is attributed to its cell membrane, composed of two external lipid layers, which has been touted to possess stronger antioxidant abilities than vitamin E [22].

Few studies exist to confirm the topical effect of astaxanthin [23], but it has been studied extensively as an oral supplement [24]. Astaxanthin in concentrations of 0.03–0.07% produces a pink-colored cream. This limits the concentration that can be used, but no topical adverse reactions have been associated with this carotenoid. The topical antioxidant benefits of astaxanthin have not been established.

Lutein

Another carotenoid found in topical cosmeceuticals is lutein. It is naturally found in green leafy vegetables, such as spinach and kale. Lutein is an antioxidant in the plant kingdom, also being used for blue light absorption. In the animal kingdom, lutein is found in egg yolks, animal fats, and the corpus luteum. It is a lipophilic molecule, not soluble in water, characterized by a long polyene side chain composed of conjugated double bonds. These double bonds are degraded by light and heat, a universal characteristic of carotenoids to a greater or lesser degree [25]. The topical value of lutein in wound healing has never been evaluated.

Lycopene

Lycopene is a potent carotenoid found in most fruits and vegetables with a red color including tomatoes, watermelon, pink grapefruit, papaya, gac, red bell pepper, and pink guava. Lycopene is a highly unsaturated hydrocarbon containing 11 conjugated and two unconjugated double bonds, which makes it a longer molecule than any other carotenoid. This makes its absorption into the skin doubtful. It undergoes cis-isomerization when exposed to sunlight. Even though lycopene was the new oral supplement added to many commercial multivitamins this year, its topical value has never been documented. It is safe for skin application, but may stain the skin in high concentration.

Retinol

Of all the topical carotenoids, retinol is the best understood, since it is necessary for vision and possesses a well-characterized skin receptor [26]. Prescription retinoids, such as tazarotene and tretinoin, are well studied for their ability to induce the skin changes noted in Table 7.2, and OTC retinoids may demonstrate some of the same effects, to a lesser degree [27,28].

It is theoretically possible to interconvert the retinoids from one form to another. For example, retinyl palmitate and retinyl propionate, chemically known as retinyl esters, can become biologically active following cutaneous enzymatic cleavage of the ester bond and subsequent conversion to retinol. Retinol is the naturally occurring vitamin A form found in red, yellow, and orange fruits and vegetables. It is the pigment responsible for vision, but is highly unstable. Retinol can be oxidized to retinaldehyde and then oxidized to retinoic acid, also known as prescription tretinoin. It is this cutaneous

Table 7.2 Cutaneous effects of topical retinoids.

Gross dermatologic effects

1   Improvement in fine and coarse facial wrinkling
2   Decreased tactile roughness
3   Reduction of actinic keratoses
4   Lightening of solar lentigenes

Histologic dermatologic effects

1   Reduction in stratum corneum cohesion
2   Decreased epidermal hyperplasia
3   Increased production of collagen, elastin, and fibronectin
4   Reduction in tonofilaments, desmosomes, melanosomes
5   More numerous Langerhans cells
6   Angiogenesis
7   Decreased glycosaminoglycans
8   Reduced activity of collagenase and gelatinase
9   Normalization of keratinization of the pilosebaceous unit

conversion of retinol to retinoic acid that is responsible for the biologic activity of some of the new stabilized OTC vitamin A preparations designed to improve the appearance of benign photodamaged skin [29]. Unfortunately, only small amounts of retinyl palmitate and retinol can be converted by the skin, accounting for the increased efficacy seen with prescription preparations containing retinoic acid.

The main problem with prescription retinoids is their irritancy. Unfortunately, as the biological efficacy of the retinoid increases, so does the irritancy. This is also the case with the OTC retinoids. Retinol is more irritating than the retinyl esters and also more unstable. It is for this reason that cosmeceutical formulations not manufactured under strict oxygen-free conditions prefer to add retinyl palmitate to moisturizing creams. However, the retinyl palmitate may act as an antioxidant for the lipids present in the moisturizer.

The topical benefit of retinol has been documented by well-controlled studies [30]. It is commonly felt among dermatologists that retinol is of benefit [31], but it is difficult in moisturizer studies that do not include vehicle control to separate the retinol benefit from the moisturizer benefit. Nevertheless, of all the carotenoids available for formulation, retinol has the most evidence to support topical application efficacy following resurfacing.

Flavonoids

Flavonoids are aromatic compounds, frequently with a yellow color, that occur in higher plants. Five thousand flavonoids have been identified with a similar chemical structure, possessing 15 carbon atoms and a variety of biologic activities (Table 7.3) [32]. Flavonoids can be divided into flavones, flavonols, isoflavones, and flavanones, each with a slightly different chemical structure. Currently, the most common isoflavones incorporated into cosmeceuticals are daidzein and genistein, derived from soybeans. Other sources of flavonoids include curcumin, silymarin, pycnogenol, and gingko.

Table 7.3 Biologic activity of flavonoids.

1 Photoprotection against UVB
2 Quenching of reactive oxygen species
3 Metal chelation
4 Inhibition of targeted enzymes
5 Hormonal modulation
6 Anti-inflammatory activity
7 Microorganism growth inhibition
8 Antioxidant effect of multiple organ systems

Soy

The soybean-derived isoflavones genistein and daidzein function as phyto-estrogens when orally consumed, and have been credited with the decrease in cardiovascular disease and breast cancer seen in Asian women [33]. These isoflavones are present when the soy is fermented [34]. Some of the cutaneous effects of soy have been linked to its estrogenic effect in postmenopausal women. Topical estrogens have been shown to increase skin thickness and promote collagen synthesis [35]. It is interesting to note that genistein increases collagen gene expression in cell culture, but there are no published reports of this collagen-stimulating effect in topical human trials. Genistein has also been reported to function as a potent antioxidant, scavenging peroxyl radicals and protecting against lipid peroxidation in vivo [36]. The only studies that document the ability of soy to protect against UVB-induced skin damage are in mice, where a topical application of non-denatured soy extracts reduced UVB-induced cyclooxygenase-2 expression, prostaglandin-E2 secretion, and inhibited p38 MAP kinase activation [37].

Curcumin

Curcumin is a popular natural yellow food coloring used in everything from prepackaged snack foods to meats. It is sometimes used in skin-care products as a natural yellow coloring in products that claim to be free of artificial ingredients. Curcumin comes from the rhizome of the turmeric plant and is consumed orally as an Asian spice, frequently found in rice dishes to color the otherwise white rice yellow. However, this yellow color is undesirable in cosmetic preparations, since yellowing of products is typically associated with oxidative spoilage. Tetrahydrocurcumin, a hydro-genated form of curcumin, is off-white in color and can be added to skin-care products not only to function as a skin antioxidant but also to prevent the lipids in the moisturizer from becoming rancid. The antioxidant effect of tetrahydrocurcumin is said to be greater than vitamin E by cosmetic chemists. It is said to provide antioxidant skin benefits by quenching oxygen radicals and inhibiting nuclear factor-κB [38,39].

Silymarin

Silymarin is an extract of the milk thistle (*Silybum marianum*), which belongs to the aster family of plants including diasies, thistles, and arti-chokes. The plant is named milk thistle because the oldest recorded use of the extract was to enhance human lactation, and because the plant produces a white milky sap. The extract consists of three flavinoids derived from the fruit, seeds, and leaves of the plant. These flavonoids are silybin, silydianin, and silychristin. Homeopathically, silymarin is used to treat liver disease, but it is a strong antioxidant, preventing lipid peroxidation by scavenging free radical species. Its antioxidant effects have been demonstrated topically in hairless mice by a 92% reduction in skin tumors following UVB exposure [40,41]. The mechanism for this decrease in tumor production is unknown, but topical silymarin has been shown to decrease the formation of pyrimidine dimers in a mouse model [42]. It has also been found to improve the healing of burns in albino rats [43], which is the rationale for its incorporation into some wound-healing and post-resurfacing preparations.

Silymarin is found in a number of high-end moisturizers for benign photoaging to prevent cutaneous oxidative damage and to reduce facial redness. A double-blind placebo-controlled study in 46 subjects with stage I–III rosacea found improvement in skin redness, papules, itching, hydration, and skin color [44]. This was felt to be due to its direct activity on modulating cytokines and angiokines.

Pycnogenol

Pycnogenol is an extract of French marine pine bark (*Pinus pinaster*). The extract is a water-soluble liquid containing several phenolic constituents, including taxifolin, catechin, procyanidins. It also contains several phenolic acids, including p-hydroxybenzoic, protocatechuic, gallic, vanillic, p-couric, caffeic, and ferulic. It is a trademarked ingredient, a potent free radical scavenger that can reduce the vitamin C radical, returning the vitamin C to its active form (VI,C) [45]. The active vitamin C in turn regenerates vitamin E to its active form, maintaining the natural oxygen-scavenging mechanisms of the skin intact.

Pycnogenol is the ideal anti-aging additive since it demonstrates no chronic toxicity, no mutagenicity, no teratogenicity, and no allergenicity [46]. In B16 melanoma cells, it was shown to inhibit tyrosinase activity and melanin biosynthesis [47]. Many discussions of antioxidant flavonoids include a mention of pycnogenol, but few high-quality data are presented [48].

Ginkgo

Ginkgo biloba, also named the maidenhair tree, is the last member of the Ginkgoaceae family, which grew on earth some 200–250 million years ago. For this reason, ginkgo contains flavonoids not found in other botanicals. It possesses bilobalide (a sequiterpene), ginkgolides (diterpenes with 20 carbon atoms), and other aromatic substances such as ginkgol, bilobdol, and ginkgolic acid. It is a plant with numerous purported benefits and has been a common part of homeopathic medicine in East Asia for 4000 years. The plant leaves are said to contain unique polyphenols such as terpenoids (ginkgolides, bilobalides), flavinoids, and flavonol glycosides that have anti-inflammatory effects. These anti-inflammatory effects have been linked to anti-radical and anti-lipoperoxidant effects in experimental fibroblast models [49]. Ginkgo flavonoid fractions containing quercetin, kaempferol, sciadopitysin, ginkgetin, and isoginkgetin have been demonstrated to induce human skin fibroblast proliferation in vitro. Increased collagen and extracellular fibronectin were also demonstrated by radioisotope assay [50]. Ginkgo extracts are therefore added to many cosmeceuticals to function as antioxidants and promoters of collagen synthesis following resurfacing, based on non-human models of oxidative damage.

Polyphenols

Polyphenols are a subset of flavonoids used in many cosmeceuticals. Two main sources of polyphenols are teas and fruits. This section presents green tea and pomegranate as examples of the evidence available to support polyphenol biologic activity.

Green tea

Tea (*Camellia sinensis*) is botanical popular in East Asia for 5000 years, used both topically and orally. There are several different types of teas: green, black, oolong, and white. The different teas come from the same plant, but different processing imparts different properties. Green tea is made from unfermented tea leaves and contains the highest concentration of polyphenol antioxidants [51]. Black tea leaves are fermented for some days before heating. Oolong tea originates in the Fujian province of China and the leaves are treated much like black tea, except that the withering and fermentation times are minimized. White tea comes from young tea leaves that are harvested for a few days each spring when the plant emerges from the ground. These leaves are said to be very high in antioxidants. The highest-quality white tea is obtained from buds that are just ready to open, known as needles or tips.

Green tea is manufactured from both the leaf and the bud of the plant. Orally, green tea is said to contain beneficial polyphenols, such as epicatechin, epicatechin-3-gallate, epigallocatechin, and epigallocatechin-3-gallate (EGCG), which function as potent antioxidants [52]. EGCG is the most potent of the polyphenols, and it is sold as a white caffeine-free powder [53]. Other alkaloids present in green tea include caffeine, theobromine, and theophylline.

Green tea can be easily added to topical creams and lotions designed to combat the signs of photoaging, but it must be stabilized itself with an antioxidant, such as butylated hydroxytoluene. The Mayo Clinic Drugs and Supplements rates the evidence to support green tea as a photoprotectant as a C [54].

A study by Katiyar *et al.* demonstrated the anti-inflammatory effects of topical green tea application on C3H mice. A topically applied green tea extract containing GTP ((-)-epigallocatechin-3-gallate) was found to reduce UVB-induced inflammation as measured by double skin-fold swelling [55]. They also found protection against UV-induced edema, erythema, and antioxidant depletion in the epidermis. This was further investigated by applying GTP to the back of humans 30 minutes prior to UV irradiation, which resulted in decreased myeloperoxidase activity and decreased infiltration of leukocytes as compared to untreated skin [56].

The application of topical green tea polyphenols prior to UV exposure has also been shown to decrease the formation of cyclobutane pyrimidine dimers [57]. These dimers are critical in initiating UV-induced mutagenesis and carcinogenesis, which represent the end stage of the aging process. Thus, green tea polyphenols can function topically as antioxidants, anti-inflammatories, and anti-carcinogens, making them a popular cosmeceutical additive [58,59].

Pomegranate

Pomegranate (*Punica granatum*) is a deciduous tree bearing a red fruit native to Afghanistan, Pakistan, Iran, and northern India [60]. It was brought to California by the Spanish settlers in 1769 and is commercially cultivated for its juice. Pomegranate juice, commonly consumed in the Middle East, provides about 16% of the adult requirement of vitamin C per 100 mg serving. It also contains pantothenic acid, also known as vitamin B5, potassium, and antioxidant polyphenols. These substances have been demonstrated to protect against UVA- and UVB-induced cell damage in SKU-1064 human skin fibroblasts [61]. Pomegranate juice has also been purported to reduce oxidative stress and to affect low-density lipoprotein (LDL) and platelet aggregation in humans and apolipoprotein E-deficient mice [62,63]. It has also been studied for improving hyperlipidemia in diabetic patients [64]. It is found in some wound-healing preparations to promote healing, but its value has never been demonstrated.

Other antioxidants used in post-resurfacing formulations

Other antioxidants are commonly found in commercial preparations for use after resurfacing procedures. These ingredients are used to promote healing, and they include aloe vera and ubiquinone.

Aloe vera

Probably the most widely used cutaneous botanical anti-inflammatory is aloe vera. The mucilage is released from the plant leaves as a colorless gel containing 99.5% water and a complex mixture of mucopolysaccharides,

20 Halder RM, Richards GM. Management of dyschromias in ethnic skin. *Dermatol Ther* 2004; **17**: 151–7.

21 Hussein G, Sankawa U, Goto H, Matsumoto K, Watanabe H. Astaxanthin, a carotenoid with potential in human health and nutrition. *J Nat Prod* 2006; **69**: 443–9.

22 Karppi J, Rissanen TH, Nyyssonen K, et al. Effects of astaxanthin supplementation of lipid peroxidation. *Int J Vitam Nutr Res* 2007; **77**: 3–11.

23 Seki T. Effects of astaxanthin on human skin. *Fragrance J* 2001; **12**: 98–103.

24 Higuera-Ciapara I, Felix-Valenzuela L, Goycoolea FM. Astaxanthin: a review of its chemistry and applications. *Crit Rev Food Sci Nutr* 2006; **46**: 185–96.

25 Alves-Rodrigues A, Shao A. The science behind lutein. **Toxicol Lett** 2004; **150**: 57–83.

26 Kligman LH, Do CH, Kligman AM. Topical retinoic acid enhances the repair of ultraviolet damaged dermal connective tissue. *Connect Tissue Res* 1984; **12**: 139–50.

27 Goodman DS. Vitamin A and retinoids in health and disease. *N Eng J Med* 1984; **310**: 1023–31.

28 Noy N. Interactions of retinoids with lipid bilayers and with membranes. In: Livrea MA, Packer L, eds., *Retinoids*. New York, NY: Marcel Dekker, 1993, pp. 17–27.

29 Duell EA, Derguini F, Kang S, Elder JT, Voorhees JJ. Extraction of human epidermis treated with retinol yields retro-retinoids in addition to free retinol and retinyl esters. *J Invest Dermatol* 1996; **107**: 178–82.

30 Kafi R, Swak HS, Schumacher WE, et al. Improvement of naturally aged skin with vitamin A (retinol). *Arch Dermatol* 2007; **143**: 606–12.

31 Hruza GJ. Retinol benefits naturally aged skin. *J Watch Dermatol* 2007 June.

32 Arct J, Pytokowska K. Flavonoids as components of biologically active cosmeceuticals. *Clin Dermatol* 2008; **26**: 347–57.

33 Glazier MG, Bowman MA. A review of the evidence for the use of phytoestrogens as a replacement for traditional estrogen replacement therapy. *Arch Intern Med* 2001; **161**: 1161–72.

34 Friedman M, Brandon DL. Nutritional and health benefits of soy proteins. *J Agric Food Chem* 2001; **49**: 1069–86.

35 Maheux R, Naud F, Rioux M, et al. A randomized, double-blind, placebo-controlled study on the effect of conjugated estrogens on skin thickness. *Am J Obset Gynecol* 1994; **170**: 642–9.

36 Wiseman H, O'Reilly JD, Adlercreutz H, et al. Isoflavone phytoestrogens consumed in soy decrease F-2-isoprostane concentrations and increase resistance of low-density lipoprotein to oxidation in humans. *Am J Clin Nutr* 2000; **72**: 395–400.

37 Chen N, Scarpa R, Zhang L, Seiberg M, Lin CB. Nondenatured soy extracts reduce UVB-induced skin damage via multiple mechanisms. *Photochem Photobiol* 2008; **84**: 1551–9.

38 Hatcher H, Planalp R, Cho J, Torti FM, Torti SV. Curcumin: from ancient medicine to current clinical trials. *Cell Mol Life Sci* 2008; **65**: 1631–52.

39 Jagetia GC, Aggarwal BB. "Spicing up" of the immune system by curcumin. *J Clin Immunol* 2007; **27**: 19–35.

40 Katiyar SK, Korman NJ, Mukhtar H, Agarwal R. Protective effects of silymarin against photocarcinogenesis in a mouse skin model. *J Natl Cancer Inst* 1997; **89**: 556–66.

41 Katiyar SK. Silymarin and skin cancer prevention: anti-inflammatory, antioxidant and immunomodulatory effects. *Int J Oncol* 2005; **26**: 169–76.

42 Chatterjee L, Agarwal R, Mukhtar H. Ultraviolet B radiation-induced DNA lesions in mouse epidermis: an assessment sing a novel 32P-postlabeling technique. *Biochem Biophys Res Commun* 1996; **229**: 590–5.

43 Toklu HZ, Tunali-Akbay T, Erkanli G, Yuksel M, Ercan F, Sener G. Silymarin, the antioxidant component of *Silybum marianum*, protects against burn-induced oxidative skin injury. *Burns* 2007; **33**: 908–16.

44 Berardesca E, Cameli N, Cavallotti C, Levy JL, Pierard GE, de Paoli Ambrosi G. Combined effects of silymarin and methyisulfonylmethane in the managementof rosacea: clinical and instrumental evaluation. *J Cosmet Dermatol* 2008; **7**: 8–14.

45 Cossins E, Lee R, Packer L. ESR studies of vitamin C regeneration, order of reactivity of natural source phytochemical preparations. *Biochem Mol Biol Int* 1998; **45**: 583–98.

46 Schonlau F. The cosmetic pycnogenol. *J Appl Cosmetol* 2002; **20**: 241–6.

47 Kim YJ, Kang KS, Yokozawa T. The anti-melanogenic effect of pycnogenol by its anti-oxidative actions. *Food Chem Toxicol* 2008; **46**: 2466–71.

48 Rona C, Vailati F, Berardesca D. The cosmetic treatment of wrinkles. *J Cosmet Dermatol* 2004; **3**: 26–34.

49 Joyeux M, Lobstein A, Anton R, Mortier F. Comparative antilipoperoxidant, antinecrotic and scavenging properties of terpenes and biflavones from Ginkgo and some flavonoids. *Plant Med* 1995; **61**: 126–9.

50 Kim SJ, Lim MH, Chun IK, Won YH. Effects of flavonoids of Ginkgo biloba on proliferation of human skin fibroblast. *Skin Pharmacol* 1997; **10**: 200–5.

51 Hsu S. Green tea and the skin. *J Am Acad Dermatol* 2005; **52**: 1049–59.

52 Katiyar SK, Elmets CA. Green tea and skin. *Arch Dermatol* 2000; **136**: 989–94.

53 Geria NM. Green, black or white, it fits beauty to a "t". *HAPPI* December 2006: 46–50.

54 Chui AD, Chan JL, Kern DG, *et al*. Double-blinded, placebo-controlled trial of green tea extracts in the clinical and histologic appearance of photoaging skin. *Dermatol Surg* 2005; **31**: 855–60.

55 Katiyar SK, Elmets CA, Agarwal R, *et al*. Protection against ultraviolet-B radiation-induced local and systemic suppression of contact hypersensitivity and edema responses in C3H/HeN mice by green tea polyphenols. *Photochem Photobiol* 1995; **62**: 855–61.

56 Elmets CA, Singh D, Tubesing K, Matsui MS, Katiyar SK, Mukhtar H. Green tea polyphenols as chemopreventive agents against cutaneous photodamage. *J Am Acad Dermatol* 2001; **44**: 425–32.

57 Katiyar SK, Afaq F, Perez A, Mukhtar H. Green tea polyphenol treatment to human skin prevents formation of ultraviolet light B-induced pyrimidine dimers in DNA. *Clin Cancer Res* 2000; **6**: 3864–9.

58 Ahmad N, Mukhtar H. Cutaneous photochemoprotection by green tea: a brief review. *Skin Pharmacol Appl Skin Physiol* 2001; **14**: 69–76.

59 Mukhtar H, Katiyar SK, Agarwal R. Green tea and skin: anticarcinogenic effects. *J Invest Dermatol* 1994; **102**: 3–7.

60 Jurenka JS. Therapeutic applications of pomegranate (*Punica granatum* L.): a review. *Altern Med Rev* 2008; **13**: 128–44.

61 Pacheco-Palencia LA, Noratto G, Hingorani L, Talcott ST, Mertens-Talcott SU. Protective effects of standardized pomegranate (Punica granatum L.) polyphenolic extract in ultraviolet-irradiated human skin fibroblasts. *J Agric Food Chem* 2008; **56**: 8434–41.

62 Aviram M, Rosenblat M, Gaitini D, *et al*. Pomegranate juice consumption for 3 years by patients with carotid artery stenosis reduces common carotid intima-media thickness, blood pressure and LDL oxidation. *Clin Nutr* 2004; **23**: 423–33.

63 Aviram M, Dornfeld L, Rosenblat M, *et al*. Pomegranate juice consumption reduces oxidative stress, atherogenic modifications to LDL, and platelet aggregation: studies in humans and in atherosclerotic apolipoprotein e-deficient mice. *Am Journ Clin Nutr* 2000; **71**: 1062–76.

64 Esmaillzadeh A, Tahbaz F, Gaieni I, Alavi-Majd H, Azadbakht L. Concentrated pomegranate juice improves profiles in diabetic patients with hyperlipidemia. *J Med Food* 2004; **7**: 305–8.

65 McKeown E. Aloe vera. *Cosmet Toilet* 1987; **102**: 64–5.

66 Waller T. Aloe vera. *Cosmet Toilet* 1992; **107**: 53–4.

67 Maenthaisong R, Chaiyakunapruk N, Niruntraporn S. Kongkaew C. The efficacy of aloe vera for burn wound healing: a systematic review. *Burns* 2007; **33**: 713–18.

68 Orafidiya LO, Agbani EO, Oyedele AO, Babalola OO, Onayemi O, Aiyedun FF. The effect of aloe vera gel on the anti-acne properties of the essential iol of *Ocimum gratissimum* Linn leaf: a preliminary clinical investigation. *Int J Aromather* 2004; **14**: 15–21.

69 Puvabanditsin P, Vongtongsri R. Efficacy of aloe vera cream in prevention and treatment of sunburn and suntan. *J Med Assoc Thai* 2005; **88:** S173–6.

70 Reuter J, Jocher A, Stump J, Grossjohann B, Franke G, Sshempp CM. Investigation of the anti-inflammatory potential of Aloe vera gel (97.5%) in the ultraviolet erythema test. *Skin Pharmacol Physiol* 2008; **21**: 106–10.

71 Hoppe U, Bergemann J, Diembeck W, *et al.* Coenzyme Q10, a cutaneous antioxidant and energizer. *Biofactors* 1999; **9**: 371–8.

72 Blatt T, Mundt C, Mummert C, *et al.* Modulation of oxidative stresses in human aging skin. *Z Gerontol Geriatr* 1999; **32**: 83–8.

73 Sohal RS, Kamzalov S, Sumien N, *et al.* Effect of coenzyme Q10 intake on endogenous coenzyme Q content, mitrochondrial electron transport chain, antioxidant defenses, and life span of mice. *Free Radic Biol Med* 2006; **40**: 480–7.

74 Passi S, De Pita O, Grandinetti M, Simotti C, Littarru GP. The combined use of oral and topical lipophilic antioxidants increases their levels both in sebum and stratum corneum. *Biofactors* 2003; **18**: 289–97.

75 Fuller B, Smith D, Howerton A, Kern D. Anti-inflammatory effects of coQ10 and colorless carotenoids. *J Cosmet Dermatol* 2006; **5**: 30–8.

Index

Page numbers in *italics* represent figures, those in **bold** represent tables.